Your Appetite Switch

Master Your Eating & Free Your Life

Anne Katherine, MA, CEDS

©2010 Anne Katherine
All Rights Reserved
Printed in the United States of America

No part of this publication may be reproduced, stored in a retrieval system, or transmitted, in any form, or by any means, electronic, mechanical, photocopying, recording, or otherwise, without the written permission of the author, except in the case of brief quotations embodied in reviews or reports, or derivations in any type of media, and these must be cited, including the name, Anne Katherine, and the title, *Your Appetite Switch*. For information, address Anne Katherine, Box 538, Coupeville, WA 98239, call 206-527-5492, or write compass@whidbey.net.

www.annekatherine.org
or
www.masteryourappetite.com

ISBN: 1452884307
EAN-13: 9781452884301

Endorsements

During the last hundred years or so there have been more than a **dozen important discoveries** in health care made by individual therapists who were not employed by a university, hospital or other research organization, some by doctors of the three major professions but some by other therapists. Usually these discoveries are the result of observation, frustration, lateral thinking and individual research. Few received much media attention and the information was under-utilized. Potential benefits were unavailable to the majority.

The **APPETITE SWITCH is one of these discoveries**.

If you are fortunate enough to read this you have the opportunity to be one of those to benefit from a discovery that may not make the headlines. The author describes the physical, chemical, neurological and psychological aspects of problems relating to eating too much or unwisely. Then she presents **an effective plan that you CAN follow**.

It is well written and easy to understand. Anne Katherine understands that order and timing are important; that psychological change must come before physical change. This alone places her plan above any other you may have tried.

Dr. Glenn Smead, DC
Alternative Medicine Practitioner including Thought Field Therapy, Applied Physiology and some aspects of Chinese medicine, for over 50 years. Jefferson City, Mo

"Small steps are important when you've made hundreds of efforts that haven't worked!" (page 4) This seems so obvious and yet so wise. What Anne Katherine is doing in *Your Appetite Switch* is continuing her remarkable and unyielding march into uncharted territory—the Brain.

Here she makes the (sometimes) lifelong battles fought by millions of overeaters progressively understandable. The real battle is in the reactions inside our brains.

In *Your Appetite Switch*, Katherine shows us how to "unstick" the switch by interrupting the brain's chain reactions in an **incredibly satisfying series of small and - believe me on this- EASY steps.**

Yes, I know every diet promises "easy" but they do so by leaving out common sense steps and substituting often extreme solutions. *Your Appetite Switch* won't let you get away with skipping the important stuff...in fact, Anne Katherine makes it almost impossible NOT to do the necessary actions that will yield **long term, effective, life changing**, and make-no-mistake serious weight loss!

In fact this program addresses changes that will transform more than weight. You will be more relaxed, more in control of personal choices, and mentally, as well as physically, healthier!

Sherry Buckner
Therapist, Consultant, Facilitator, Denver, Colorado

In this well researched book, Anne Katherine applies **30 years of brain chemistry research** to the real reasons why some of us eat too much and cannot stop. She helps us understand the effect of food on the brain cells, and body cells, and she puts the scientific information into a form we can understand and apply. If you've struggled with food, and with how to get control of your eating behavior, *YOUR APPETITE SWITCH* will lead you to the **right solution for you**. Calm and compassionate, this book is a must read for people who struggle endlessly with food, eating and body weight.

H. Theresa Wright, MS, RD, LDN
Renaissance Nutrition Center, Inc., East Norriton, Pennsylvania

If this book had been written 30 years ago and I had taken its suggestions, I might have been able to recover from my food addiction before I had to do two in-patient treatments and three months in a halfway house for food addiction. I hope this book reaches a large audience of newly suffering food addicts and the professionals who serve them."

Mary Foushi
Executive Director of ACORN Food Dependency Recovery Services, Sarasota, Florida
Author of *Food Addiction Recovery: A New Model for Professional Support.*
(Mary has been abstinent from her addictive foods for over 20 years and has maintained a 195 pound weight loss.)

Anne Katherine's groundbreaking book, *Anatomy of a Food Addiction: The Brain Chemistry of Overeating* brought the basics of chemical dependency therapy for food to the general public. In *Your Appetite Switch*, Katherine brings the advances in science and treatment of the last two decades to an even wider readership. A **delight to read**, Katherine's newest book takes the often complicated process of recovering from food addiction and breaks it down to **one single, doable weekly action**, all the while maintaining a **light, often humorous,** spiritual perspective.

Philip R. Werdell, MA
Chair of the Food Addiction Institute, Sarasota, Florida
Author of *Bariatric Surgery and Food Addiction.*

I have had the privilege of working with Anne in her transition from educator, clinician, to author. *Your Appetite Switch* is her latest accomplishment in combining all those roles. Anne Katherine is that rare clinician author whose published works over the years always pushes the "knowledge envelope" for the reader to unlock "their personal unknown," in this case, care for their body. To create true self-help, an author must have the capacity to form a link with the reader. Anne Katherine masterfully accomplishes that task in *Your Appetite Switch*.

Lt. Col. Bert Bauer, LCSW, (Army Ret.)
Author of *A Failed State in Buckhead* (To be in print in 2011)
Military Consultant for Front Line emotional support, North Georgia

Also by Anne Katherine

Boundaries, Where You End and I Begin

Anatomy of a Food Addiction

Where to Draw the Line

When Misery is Company

How to Make Almost Any Diet Work

Lick It! Fix Her Appetite Switch

Penumbra, Book 1. Lifetimes of a Soul

Dedicated to Rabbitt and Cliff Boyer
For saving our collective posteriors above and beyond . . .

Awed Gratitude to my Incredible Friends & Support Team
Being one who prefers to handle problems on my own,
who much prefers being the helper, rather than the helpee,
I am humbled by the attentiveness, generosity, spontaneous showing-up,
and all-round integrity of my friends during a challenging time.
You keep my core going. Thank you!

Sherry Ascher
Shirley Averett
Sherry Buckner
Claudia Byram
Marilyn Clay
Scott Edelstein
Joan and Blaine Haigh
Susan Johnson
Lynn and Rick Keat
Harry Lynam and Barbara Self
Jean Malpas
Karen Selby
Jill and Kevin Shea
Linda Stafford
Tom and Susanne Stein
Frances West
Ann Briel Weston
Connie Wolfe
Mary Zibung

When the going gets arduous, true friends get ardent.

Warning!

This book will change your eating.

Please check with your doctor to see if a change in food choices and decreased intake will affect you or your medications in a way that should be monitored.

If your doctors want to support you and not say inadvertent comments that will sabotage you, urge them to read *Lick It! Fix Her Appetite Switch* by Anne Katherine

Table of Contents

1. Your Appetite Switch — 1
2. Rule 2 — 6
3. Training Week — 10
4. Training Week, Day 1 — 17
5. Training Week, Day 2 — 22
6. First Challenge — 25
7. Preparing for Day 3 — 27
8. Day 3 — 45
9. Getting Ready for Day 4 — 51
10. Training Week, Day 4 — 56
11. Training Week, Day 5 — 62
12. Day 6 — 66
13. Training Week, Last Day — 70
14. Week 1, Test 1 — 84
15. The First Weekend after Training Week, Day 6 — 95
16. The Battle in the Brain — 105
17. Meanwhile, Back at the Testing Center — 111
18. Preparing for Test 2 — 114
19. Week 2, Test 2 — 118
20. Analyzing Data from Test 1 — 120
21. Meanwhile, Back at Test 2 — 122
22. The Magic Pill — 124
23. Week 3, Test 3 — 134
24. Homesick? — 137
25. Week 4, The Seduction of Stress — 144
26. The Wall — 158

27	*Maintaining Mastery of Your Appetite Switch*	*182*
A	*What Next?*	*185*
B	*Analyzing Test 1*	*188*
C	*Analysis of Test 2*	*203*
D	*Analysis of Test 3*	*212*
E	*Analysis of Test 5*	*223*
F	*Resources*	*226*
G	*Index*	*229*
	About Anne Katherine	*232*

1 Your Appetite Switch

In your brain, you have a switch. It turns on and off. When it's on, you want to eat.

When you want to eat too much, your appetite switch is stuck. It's not turning off when it should. We can fix this problem.

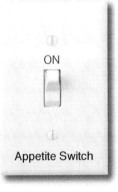
Appetite Switch

If you are willing to make five changes, you can master your appetite. In fact, your appetite will stop driving you crazy within one month if you will make just three changes, but there are some rules.

The first rule is: take each test, each change, and each chapter in order. What you have in this book is a tool that will work miraculously if you will use it exactly as designed. Each person who has followed this plan has felt joyous relief as her appetite stopped nagging her.

Abbe came into this program after 50 failed diets. She swore that she'd tried every major diet that had hit the checkout stands since she was fifteen. She'd eaten bananas like a baboon. She'd swallowed protein drinks with the delicious taste of fermented bouillon. She'd eaten raw, liquid, and color-coordinated meals.

> **Rule 1.**
> Take each test and each chapter in order.

She'd actually given up on dieting long ago, but now she was worried. Her blood tests were showing cholesterol levels that were endangering her. She knew that the statistics were against her. Well past middle age, she was afraid it was too late, that her body was so entrenched that it would not respond to a different way of eating.

She'd also lost faith in her own ability to change.

I started her out exactly as I'm starting you, and in three weeks, her appetite showed a verifiable shift. Not only could she feel and see a difference, the records she kept proved her appetite switch was turning itself off. When her cholesterol dropped 50 points, she had further proof.

You can see similar results for yourself. In three weeks, you can prove to yourself that your appetite switch is being repaired.

You will give yourself 5 tests.

Each week, for five weeks, you will give yourself one test, five tests in all. Each test will have an effect on one brain chemical or one brain process that influences the appetite switch.

At the end of each week, you'll look at your test results. If a test decreases your appetite, then you'll know the chemical tested has been an important factor in your eating.

When a test is successful in the sense of turning off your appetite switch, you will then convert it into a change. By making that change, you can master your appetite.

How this book will work for you.

The testing period will last six weeks. At the end of six weeks, you will have made as many as five changes, and balanced the major players in your stuck appetite switch.

The first week will be a Training Week. Each day you'll learn and practice one research tool. At the end of the Training Week, you'll have the tools you'll use to research your appetite switch.

You'll have options about how much data you want to gather on each test. You can harvest a lot of information or a minimal amount. It's your choice.

Either way, the process will work. If you choose to stop collecting data or if you don't want to interpret the results, that's OK. You may have to keep the tests going longer than five weeks to see the results, but the system itself will still work, turning off your appetite switch.

No Skipping

Don't skip ahead now. The tests are listed in a particular order on purpose. Any test that is converted into a change makes later ones easier. In fact, many books and programs make the mistake of starting people on a change before they've had adequate preparation for it (or even before they know whether or not a particular change is necessary for them).

If you feel like skipping ahead, ask yourself:
1. Is this what I've done before?
2. Did it work then?
3. Is this a pattern of mine?
4. Does it usually help me or hurt me?
5. Could I try a different pattern and see if the outcome improves?

If you've ever been on a diet, the odds are that you were told to change something before your body was ready for it. We are going to prepare your body for each change so that it feels like a manageable step instead of a very steep step. Small steps are important when you've made hundreds of efforts that haven't worked.

Dominique wanted to push herself, a holdover from her long-time pattern of trying to force her body into submission. She wanted to skip tests and race ahead. She expected to have to call on will power to make herself stop eating, but instead she used her will power to *keep herself from skipping ahead.* By taking each test in order and fully preparing for each change, she protected herself from another failure. She got her body ready for the changes down the line.

Venetta had battled her weight her whole life. She had promised herself she would eat differently about ten thousand times. Every time she went back on a promise, she blamed herself. She had zero faith that she could ever change her eating, but within two weeks, her tests proved to her that her appetite switch was turning off.

Overeating is a chemical problem.

Imbalanced body chemicals make you overeat. We are going to rebalance your chemicals one at a time. Each time one of your chemicals gets balanced, your body will breathe a sigh of relief.

You and your body have been working against each other for a long time probably. Your body has been laboring under the chemicals that drive eating, and you've been mad at it for making you eat when you didn't want to.

You've thought less of your body, because it wouldn't do what you wanted it to, while your body was helplessly following the programming that made you reach for foods that hurt you. It's been a vicious circle and now you can stop it.

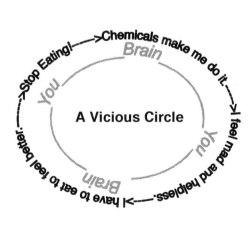

Until now, the great likelihood is that *you've been treating your body in a way that made it eat more*—not on purpose, but from persistent cultural ideas that misdirected you, and also from a combination of hopelessness and anger toward yourself.

Your body is innocent. So are you. You've done the best you could considering the deluge of misinformation that comes toward you daily. Even the experts contradict each other, but they usually agree on one point—that to have successful long-term weight loss, a person has to change her eating.

> **You've been treating your body in a way that made it eat more.**

We already know—that's a lot harder than it sounds. And one thing that makes it hard is not knowing what changes are most important and which changes should go first.

Change your eating—good idea, but how? Not because someone says to, but because you can see, within a maximum of three weeks, that a change is making you feel different and helping you to eat differently.

Imagine, choosing smaller portions at dinner, not because you're gritting your teeth and forcing yourself away from the table, but because you've lost interest in eating and want to do something else.

Imagine—what would you do with your time and energy if you weren't preoccupied with eating and feeling bad about yourself? What would you do with your life if you and your body were loving partners?

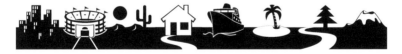

What will you do with your life when you and your body are loving partners?

2 Rule 2

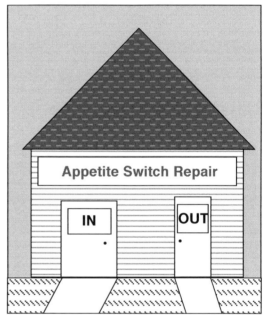

Don't change anything about your eating—yet.

We have to take into account that you've lost faith in your body. The two of you have been opponents for too long, wrestling with each other, using force and punishment, and hurting each other.

Throw yourself into the Training Week so that you'll have **data that proves your appetite switch is getting turned off.** If you are like 99% of my clients, you have a biased perspective on your body. You tend to think it is defective or flawed.

I work with groups online and in my most recent group, every single woman believed that her body was not cooperating until we analyzed her tests. In every case, test results showed an improvement in each woman's appetite switch after only one week of testing and a dramatic improvement after the second test.

So, each woman believed her body was still operating the same old way. And each week, her tests showed that her appetite switch was getting turned off.

Esther had so little faith in her body that she had a hard time doing the research. She had given up on her body years ago and thought, "What's the use? Nothing can work." Despite this, the records she did keep showed an unmistakable improvement in her chemical functioning.

I'm betting that you are climbing the same mountain, that a part of you has also lost faith and will need some hard facts to change your beliefs about yourself. Therefore the Training Week will teach you a way to track your appetite so that you'll have physical, verifiable proof that your body is cooperating with you.

> **Your *after* picture will mean much more if you have an accurate *before* picture.**

Old Ideas

Most people, encouraged as they start this program, begin to immediately change their eating in the way they think I'm going to advise later. So hold on, let's think about this.

Your head is full of ideas about what you're supposed to do to lose weight, right? You've already tried each of these ideas at least once, right? Could you sustain those practices?

I don't think so, or you wouldn't need this book. So if you go merrily forward, following your favorite old ideas, is this likely to work?

Do you think there's a remote possibility that I'm going to give you some advice that differs from some of your old ideas?

Indeed, I'm already giving you counsel contrary to one of your thoughts. You think you should change something right now, and I'm telling you to not change anything.

> **Don't change your eating today.**

If you start changing things right now, it's likely that you will either change something that your body is not ready for or that will work against fixing your appetite switch. Not only that, you'll cheat yourself of having hard data about how your switch is working today, right now.

And this will defraud you from knowing exactly how much your brain is improving and which changes make the most difference to your appetite switch.

We need to know how your switch is working *right now*, before any tests are made. Overeating is a chemical problem and we want to know which of your chemicals are making you eat.

There are no blood tests and no urine tests that will answer this question. What you *can* do is put your body through five simple tests and that will show us what changes will sustain your mastery over your appetite.

Your brain isn't like anyone else's. You may have all eleven imbalances that cause a faulty appetite switch, or you may just have three of them.

(You don't have to test all eleven. Some are part of a chain reaction, so if you eliminate one link in the chain, you eliminate the entire reaction that would otherwise force you to eat.)

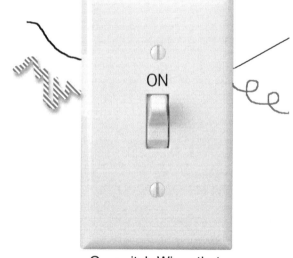

On-switch Wires that can cause Trouble

By keeping good records, you'll know exactly which chemicals are out of whack in your own head. You'll fix those and only those and know exactly what your ongoing program should be.

Imagine—instead of shooting into the dark with a one-size-does-*not*-fit-all diet, you can have a precise plan that *always* works for you. So, please, do:

- ✧ Find some patience.
- ✧ Promise yourself you'll continue to eat exactly as you've been eating.
- ✧ Eight days from now, you can take the first test.

3 Training Week

Today

Tomorrow you'll begin keeping records that you'll use to see how your body reacts to the tests you start next week. Today you'll learn to use one tool to measure your appetite switch.

This is an important week for you, because you'll be learning to be a researcher. You'll also be gathering the data that you'll compare to the results of the five tests.

About half of the women I've worked with liked learning the tools because it helped them be more conscious of what they were doing, and about half of the women hated learning the tools because it made them more conscious of what they were doing.

The ones who liked using the tools enjoyed discovering their body's patterns. They especially enjoyed seeing proof that their appetite switch was turning off.

The ones who resisted using the tools had a pattern of ignoring how they treated themselves. When they noticed their eating, they judged

> **Did you skip the last chapter and jump to this one?**
>
> If so, please go back and read chapter 2.
>
> Understanding the principles in chapter 2 will make your journey with this book *much* more effective.

themselves.

I understand that noticing yourself may go against your firm policies. So, you decide. You are at an important fork in the road.[1] I'll spell out what is down each fork, and you decide where you want to put your attention and energy.

Your Fork in the Road

Bring your energy and focus to the present.	Let your energy and focus be drawn to the past.
Approach the tests as a scientific experiment.	Treat yourself the same old punitive way.
Notice when feelings from the past start to interfere with using your research or relief tools.	Cheat yourself from collecting accurate data.
Get support for these feelings while bringing your energy and focus back to the here-and-now.	Cheat yourself from having an accurate picture of what will turn off your appetite switch.
Take the tests that will give you an accurate picture of what is keeping your appetite switch working overtime.	Continue in the old pattern of fighting yourself.
Have the information and skills you need to master your appetite.	Miss the opportunity to learn something new about yourself.

Which fork do you want to choose for right now? Be assured that I will soon give you some tools that you can use to handle feelings that would interrupt your efforts.

(If you are already having a strong reaction to the idea of looking at yourself, so that you aren't able to put aside your old pattern, you can skip to page 89 and learn a relief tool now. Come back here when you are ready.)

---

[1] Borrowed and adapted from the work of Yvonne Agazarian and Systems Centered Training and Research Institute. The full exercises/protocols are in the Systems-centered Training Manual. See www.systemscentered.com. for more information.

Watching Your Appetite—Research Tools

For all five tests, you'll measure when your appetite is pushing you and when it leaves you alone. Starting tomorrow, you'll pause each hour for less than a minute to notice how strong your appetite is. Then you will put a dot in the corresponding box for that time of day.

Any hour you are awake, notice, how intrusive is your appetite? The more intrusive your appetite is—not just thinking about a food or restaurant, but craving a particular type of food—the higher you place the dot.

For example, you might be craving something, and also want more, and also be unable to stop eating. In that case, your dot would go into the box *Can't stop eating.*

Notice the research tool below. At 7 AM, is your appetite not bothering you at all? In other words, is your attention elsewhere and not involved with food? In that case, you put a dot in the quiet row for 7:00 o'clock.

Research Tool—Appetite Measure

Training Week, Day 1		Circle Wake-up Time							
	Time of Day	5	6	7	8	9	10	11	12
	Can't stop eating								
	Want more food								
Appetite	Craving food								
	Food or restaurant focused								
	Quiet			•					

At 8:00, are you noticing that your thoughts are roaming toward a particular restaurant or food? Are food pictures floating in your head? Are you somewhat distracted from what you are doing because of food thoughts? Have you started planning, on an almost unconscious level, what

restaurant you're heading to for breakfast? Then put a dot in "Food or restaurant focused."

Basic Data--Training Week													
		Time of Day	5	6	7	8	9	10	11	12	**1**	**2**	**3**	**4**
Appetite	Can't stop eating													
	Want more food													
	Craving food													
	Food or restaurant focused					•								
	Quiet					•								

At 9:00, has the focus on food intensified into a craving? Are you now craving a particular food to the point that you are distracted from what you are supposed to be doing? You want it. You want it. You want it. In that case, put a dot into the craving food box for 9:00 am.

Basic Data--Training Week										
		Time of Day	5	6	7	8	9	10	11	12
Appetite	Can't stop eating									
	Want more food									
	Craving food								•	
	Food or restaurant focused						•			
	Quiet					•				

Barry's Chart

At 10:00, he started eating and he just wanted more. He wanted more, more, more. He put a dot in the "Want more food" box.

At 11:00, he was still eating. He couldn't stop. A dot went into the "Can't stop eating" box.

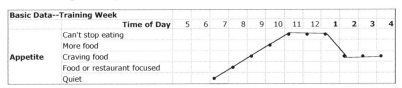

Barry continued eating through noon and 1:00 pm and then in the afternoon, he stopped eating, but food cravings continued to plague him.

At the end of the day, he drew a line through the dots so that the appetite pattern for the day was easy to see.

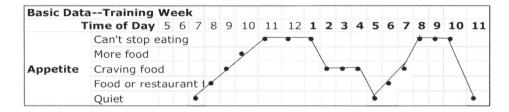

Appetite has to be noticed.

Notice that *appetite has to be noticed*, by becoming aware of your thoughts, images, and barely conscious planning. It's not felt the way hunger is felt, until it gets deeply into the craving stage, and even then, it's hard to say exactly where the craving is located. It's not felt exactly, but a craving is a powerful, almost irresistible drive toward something, and it won't be reasoned with. You can't talk yourself out of it. (Which is why you'll soon be learning how to stop the craving before it starts.)

Today's To-Do List

Today, you will prepare for tomorrow, Day 1. You have 4 tasks to do today.

1. **Make a copy** of your Basic Data Chart, Training Week, Day 1 (at the end of the chapter), unless you plan to write in this book.
2. Begin to train yourself to **pause each hour**. You can set a timer, set an alarm on your watch, phone, or computer, or notice the chimes if you are near a clock that chimes the hour.
3. Each hour, close to the top of the hour, pause and **look at your hands**. (You won't be doing anything about what you see when you look at your hands. This exercise is just to help you get used to pausing each hour.)

4. Put your Basic Data Chart **next to your bed**, so that when you wake up in the morning it will be right there for your first mark. Then take it with you the rest of the day tomorrow.

Basic Data

Tomorrow when you wake up, your first task—*even before you get out of bed*—is to notice what your appetite is doing. Is your appetite quiet or are you focused on getting some food? **Circle the time you wake up** and put a dot in the box that describes your appetite.

Frequently Asked Questions (FAQ)

Q I'm a teacher and my classes end at ten minutes to the hour. Is it OK to mark my charts 10 minutes early?

A Yes. If you have a schedule that automatically creates a pause at a certain time every hour, that's a perfect time to mark your chart. It doesn't matter if it's on the hour, on the half hour, or 10 minutes before or after the hour.

Q If I am planning to mark my chart at 10 minutes to the hour, should I put my mark in the present hour or the next hour?

A Put it in the hour you are actually in. For example, if you are marking your chart at 9:50, put your mark in the column headed by 9.

Q I got distracted. I decided to mark my charts at 8:00. 9:00. etc., but I got involved in my work and suddenly realized two hours had passed. Should I skip those hours on my chart?

A No. As soon as you remember, pause to think back to how you felt then and add those marks to your chart. (It's surprisingly difficult to remember a previous appetite intensity, so do the best you can.)

Basic Data Chart Day 1

Basic Data--Training Week, Day 1		Circle Wake-up Time	
	Time of Day	5 6 7 8 9 10 11 12 **1 2 3 4 5 6 7 8 9** 10 11 12 1 2 3 4
Appetite	Can't stop	
	Want more	
	Craving food	
	Food focused	
	Quiet	

Can't stop means you can't stop eating.

Want more means you want more food.

Craving food means you are having an urge to eat, images of food are haunting you, you are wanting a certain food, or feeling driven to get a particular type of food.

Food focused means you are partially distracted from what you are doing by thoughts of food or eating, or you might, at some level, be planning a route to a particular restaurant or planning to influence others to go to a certain restaurant.

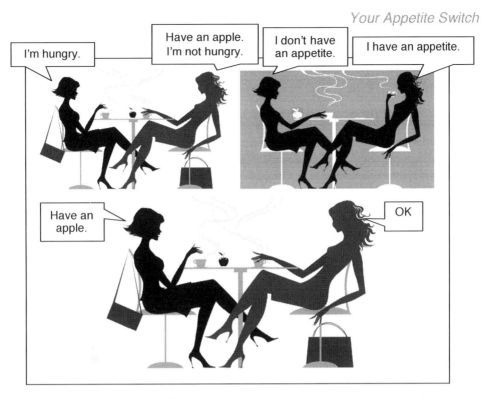

4 Training Week, Day 1

Today

1. You've already circled the time you awakened and made your first mark on your chart.
2. For the rest of the day, carry your chart with you and pause each hour to assess your appetite.
3. Put a dot at the level of appetite that most closely describes your experience at that time.
4. At the end of the day connect the dots.

(You might want to get a notebook or folder so that you can keep your charts together.)

Preparing for Day 2

Tomorrow you'll begin making a discrimination that will serve you well in the coming weeks. You'll start to notice the difference between hunger and appetite.

If you confuse the two, you're in good company. Not a week goes by that I don't see some article, quote, or comment by an educated person in which he's mixed up hunger and appetite.

Although hunger and appetite share a few of the same biochemicals and processes, for the most part they operate differently. Certain chemicals that stimulate or calm appetite have little effect on hunger.[2]

It took Cassia four weeks to begin to tell the difference between hunger and appetite, and part of the reason was that she hadn't actually been hungry for about 30 years. She'd been so driven by her appetite that she hadn't given her body a chance to be hungry.

Cravings, food pictures that frolicked in her mind, a focus on getting to certain restaurants, non-stop nibbling—these experiences kept her from noticing what was going on in her stomach.

As she learned more about herself through this program, she became aware that she feared hunger and that a part of the reason she ate almost non-stop was to prevent hunger. But the first day she noticed she was hungry, she actually laughed. Honest, basic stomach hunger turned out to be a simple and easy thing to handle.

All this eating, she then realized, was to prevent a feeling of emptiness—not from tummy-hunger—but from emotional hunger. She discovered her true fear was of being **hungry for affection or connection**. Sorting this out helped her get clear on how to respond to both issues.

If this has been all balled together for you too, we'll sort these issues

---

[2] If you're interested in the chemical breakdown, the science, and the research details of appetite versus hunger, you can find this information in one of my other books, How to Make Almost Any Diet Work. (But you're nowhere near ready to follow a diet. If you want to use that book for dieting, wait till you've completed this book.)

out, one at a time. Tomorrow, you're just doing one thing. Tomorrow you'll start noticing the difference between hunger and appetite.

Research Tool 2—Hunger Measure

Basic Data--Training Week, Day 2									Circ
	Time of Day	5	6	7	8	9	10	11	12
Hunger	Starved								
	Strong								
	Moderate								
	Mild								
	Not hungry								

As you can see, there are degrees of hunger on a continuum from not hungry at all to starving.

Each hour tomorrow, when you pause to check your appetite, you'll also notice what's going on in your stomach. Is it empty? Is your belly button rubbing up against your backbone? Are hunger pangs keeping you from thinking about anything else? Are you just a little bit hungry?

Don't work too hard at this. Just notice and put a dot at the level of hunger that most describes what you're feeling.

And **hunger *is* a feeling**, whereas **appetite is more of an urge**. Hunger is a sensation in the middle to left part of your body, near your waist. Appetite is a drive, of being compelled or pushed toward food. Hunger is sensed, and appetite is motivational, pointing you in a particular

Hunger	Appetite
Felt	Driven
Sensation	Urge
Tummy	Directed, motivational
In the body	Can be barely conscious

direction.

Today's To-Do List

1. Make a copy of the Training Week, Day 2 chart unless you are going to write in this book.
2. Put that chart next to your bed so it will be there for you to make your first marks in the morning.
3. When you wake up tomorrow, **circle the time you wake up**.
4. Notice, do you have an appetite? If so, how strong is it? Put a dot in the box that most closely describes your experience.
5. Notice, are you hungry? If so, how hungry? Put a dot in the box that comes closest to your degree of hunger.
6. Prepare to carry your chart with you throughout the day and pause each hour to assess your degrees of appetite and hunger. Put a dot at the levels of appetite and hunger that most closely describe your experience.
7. **Any time you eat anything at all, make a dot in the eating row for that hour.**
8. At the end of the day, connect the dots in each category (except eating).

FAQ

Q Can I have an appetite and not be hungry?

A Yes. You can also be hungry and not have an appetite.

Q I started eating at 8:55 and didn't finish till 9:40. Do I mark both 8 and 9?

A No. If your eating lasts for less than an hour, only mark one column. Put a dot in the box on the hour that you did most of your eating (in this case, 9:00).

Q If I mark my chart at 9:00, and I start eating at 8:50, do I record my appetite before, during, or after I eat?

A You already marked your before-meal appetite and hunger level at 8:00. Mark your appetite and hunger levels again at 9:00 or by 9:20.

Q What if I eat for 3 hours? Do I mark my eating each hour or can I just call it one meal?

A Mark your eating each hour you are eating whenever it lasts longer than one hour.

Q I just had a teeny piece of chocolate. Do I mark it?

A Yes. As teeny as it is, you are still eating.

Basic Data Chart
Day 2

Basic Data--Training Week, Day 2		Circle Wake-up Time																					
	Time of Day	5	6	7	8	9	10	11	12	1	2	3	4	5	6	7	8	9	10	11	12	1	2	3	4
Appetite	Can't stop																							
	More food																							
	Craving food																							
	Food focused																							
	Quiet																							
Hunger	Starved																							
	Strong																							
	Moderate																							
	Mild																							
	Not hungry																							
Eating	Dot																							

5 Training Week, Day 2

Today

1. Before you even get out of bed, pause and notice your levels of appetite and hunger and mark your Day 2 chart.

2. Carry your chart with you today, and pause each hour to assess and mark your degrees of hunger and appetite.

3. Put a dot in the box each hour that you eat.

4. At the end of the day, connect the dots in the hunger and appetite sections.

Preparing Your Thinking for Day 3

Jules was most challenged by Research Tool 3. This is the day she began to mark down what she was eating.

It wasn't hard for her to learn the system. As a veteran of many diets, she had no trouble knowing the difference between a carb and a protein. No, what was hard about this task was being honest about what she was eating.

She had a persistent viewpoint:

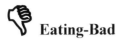

Eating-Bad   **Not eating-Good**

Plus, she liked keeping track when she thought she was eating correctly—for example, having a salad. And she didn't like keeping track when she thought she was eating incorrectly—for example, consuming ice cream.

Note that she felt this way even though I had not said a word about what she should or shouldn't be eating. (And I won't, either. You'll decide for yourself, after you have more information.)

If you have thoughts like that too—that you should be eating poached whitefish and broiled chicken breast on alternate days, along with a green salad and vinegar dressing—please pay attention. I haven't said a single word about what you should be eating, other than, **don't change your eating at all—yet**.

Remember:
- ✧ This is not about taking food away from yourself. This is about fixing a switch in your brain.
- ✧ This is not about eating, it's about the chemicals that make you eat.
- ✧ This is not a diet. It's a brain repair program.
- ✧ You will be breaking a habit—the habit of thinking that you are wrong for eating.

You have two jobs this week:
- ✧ Learn your research tools
- ✧ Begin using them.

These are your only 2 jobs. You are learning a system for tracking the symptoms of your appetite switch. You are recording how your appetite switch is working now, before you take any tests.

You are also doing something else new. You are slowing yourself down. Instead of charging forward and racing down the same blind alley you've gotten trapped by in the past, you are getting used to treating yourself differently.

Yes	No
Fixing your brain	Not taking away food
About chemicals that make you eat	Not about eating
Brain repair program	Not a diet
Breaking the habit of thinking you are wrong for eating	Not pouncing on yourself every time you eat a bite

6 First Challenge

Slow down, you're going too fast.

This is, in fact, your very first challenge, to slow yourself down and treat yourself in an entirely different way.

If you're like most of us, you rush a lot, if not outwardly, on the inside. Presented with this new system, your tendency may be to hurry up and get on with it.

You may be irritated with me for not getting right to the food and eating changes. After all, you're in a hurry—to feel better, to have a sense of getting somewhere, to feel some control, to have a better life.

Those sound like good reasons, but wait a moment, are you usually in a hurry? Are you usually racing?

Would you consider that, despite all your good reasons, being in a hurry is your pattern?

Would you also consider that being in hurry-up mode is not just about getting a lot done, but also about fleeing feelings inside of you that you are afraid to feel?

If both answers are *yes*—rushing is your pattern *and* this helps you flee from feelings you're afraid of—pause.

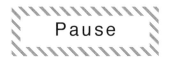
Pause

Pause and notice—is anything wrong right now?

> **Is anything wrong?**
>
> Is anything wrong in this instant,
>
> in this moment?

Pause a bit more and settle into yourself.

As you pause, consider, would you be willing to learn more about your automatic patterns? Are you curious about what you would discover if you really gave this process a chance? Are you curious about what it would be like to truly learn this process and take it step-by-step?

Are you interested in building a new relationship with yourself, one in which you actually feel better inside and out, in which you are kinder to yourself, and healthier too?

I invite you to continue to pause for 1 more minute, closing your eyes and settling more into your own center. After a minute, answer this final question.

When you paused, what did you learn or discover?

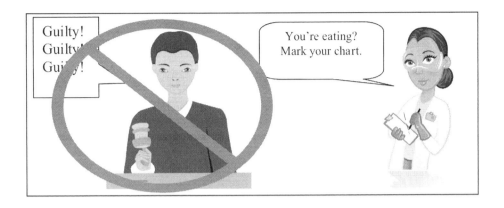

7   Preparing for Day 3

Good news! On this system:

- ❑ You won't weigh and measure your food.
- ❑ You won't have to write down the food you eat.

You will learn to see foods as chemical packages. This will enable you to record your intake rapidly and to see how your food is affecting your appetite switch.

Research Tool 3—Ingredient Tracker

This is the system you'll use to record the chemicals in the food you eat. Look at your meal as a collection of four components: protein, complex carbohydrates, simple carbs, and fat or oil.

This is good practice as you convert yourself from a Supreme Court-level punitive judge into a scientist who's looking at how her brain functions. That *is* the essential transition you are on your way to making.

You've been judging yourself for umpteen years on every bite you've put into your mouth.   We're shifting your target from your mouth to your brain, to the wires in your brain that connect to your appetite switch.

Biochemicals control the wires to your appetite switch, and chemicals are in the food you eat. As a budding scientist, you'll soon be testing the effect of food chemicals on your appetite biochemicals. And tomorrow, you'll continue to gather that all-important baseline, that control-group data, that will later show you how you've changed.

What is this?

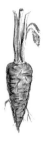

I bet you said it was a carrot.

Oh no, it is a complex carbohydrate.

And this?

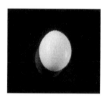

This is a protein.

How about this?

A simple carbohydrate.

And this:

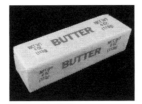

This is a fat.

To summarize, these are proteins:

These are complex carbs:

These are simple carbs:

These are fats:

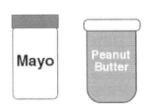

Let's practice. Identify the category. Put a dot in the box that fits.
For example:

Chicken—Where would you put the dot?

Eating	Protein		
	Complex carbohydrate		
	Simple Carbohydrate		
	Fat/oil		

Here's where it goes:

Eating	Protein	•	
	Complex carbohydrate		
	Simple Carbohydrate		
	Fat/oil		

Test yourself on these. (You are probably an expert on food composition, but another reader may not be familiar with this information.)

Fish

Eating	Protein		
	Complex carbohydrate		
	Simple Carbohydrate		
	Fat/oil		

Watermelon

Eating	Protein		
	Complex carbohydrate		
	Simple Carbohydrate		
	Fat/oil		

Banana

Eating	Protein		
	Complex carbohydrate		
	Simple Carbohydrate		
	Fat/oil		

7 Grain bread

Eating	Protein		
	Complex carbohydrate		
	Simple Carbohydrate		
	Fat/oil		

Potatoes

Eating	Protein		
	Complex carbohydrate		
	Simple Carbohydrate		
	Fat/oil		

Lettuce

Eating	Protein		
	Complex carbohydrate		
	Simple Carbohydrate		
	Fat/oil		

Lima beans

Eating	Protein		
	Complex carbohydrate		
	Simple Carbohydrate		
	Fat/oil		

Tomatoes

Eating	Protein		
	Complex carbohydrate		
	Simple Carbohydrate		
	Fat/oil		

Shrimp/Prawns

Eating	Protein		
	Complex carbohydrate		
	Simple Carbohydrate		
	Fat/oil		

Margarine

Eating	Protein	
	Complex carbohydrate	
	Simple Carbohydrate	
	Fat/oil	

Sour cream

Eating	Protein	
	Complex carbohydrate	
	Simple Carbohydrate	
	Fat/oil	

Oatmeal

Eating	Protein	
	Complex carbohydrate	
	Simple Carbohydrate	
	Fat/oil	

Popcorn

Eating	Protein	
	Complex carbohydrate	
	Simple Carbohydrate	
	Fat/oil	

I'll show you mine:

Fish

Eating	Protein	•
	Complex carbohydrate	
	Simple Carbohydrate	
	Fat/oil	

Watermelon

Eating	Protein	
	Complex carbohydrate	• F
	Simple Carbohydrate	
	Fat/oil	

Notice I did something extra with the watermelon. I added an F for fruit. Sometimes the appetite switch reacts to fruits differently than vegetables, so, just in case, I notate that.

Banana

Eating	Protein	
	Complex carbohydrate	• F
	Simple Carbohydrate	
	Fat/oil	

7 Grain bread

Eating	Protein	
	Complex carbohydrate	
	Simple Carbohydrate	•
	Fat/oil	

Most mixed grain bread has more white flour than whole-grain flour. Only 100% whole grain bread, pasta, rice, or flour gets counted as a complex carb.

Potatoes

Eating	Protein	
	Complex carbohydrate	• S
	Simple Carbohydrate	
	Fat/oil	

Here I've added an S to indicate this is a starchy vegetable, just in case that meal affects the appetite switch.

Lettuce—The *V* records that it's a vegetable, but not starchy.

Eating	Protein	
	Complex carbohydrate	•V
	Simple Carbohydrate	
	Fat/oil	

Lima beans

Eating	Protein	
	Complex carbohydrate	•S
	Simple Carbohydrate	
	Fat/oil	

Tomatoes

Eating	Protein	
	Complex carbohydrate	V•
	Simple Carbohydrate	
	Fat/oil	

Shrimp/prawns

Eating	Protein	•
	Complex carbohydrate	
	Simple Carbohydrate	
	Fat/oil	

Margarine

Eating	Protein	
	Complex carbohydrate	
	Simple Carbohydrate	
	Fat/oil	•

Sour cream

Eating	Protein	
	Complex carbohydrate	
	Simple Carbohydrate	
	Fat/oil	•

Oatmeal

Eating	Protein	
	Complex carbohydrate	•S
	Simple Carbohydrate	
	Fat/oil	

Popcorn

Eating	Protein	
	Complex carbohydrate	•S
	Simple Carbohydrate	
	Fat/oil	

For practice with more complex foods, rate these:

Buttered potatoes

Eating	Protein	
	Complex carbohydrate	
	Simple Carbohydrate	
	Fat/oil	

Fried chicken

Eating	Protein	
	Complex carbohydrate	
	Simple Carbohydrate	
	Fat/oil	

Salad with dressing

Eating	Protein	
	Complex carbohydrate	
	Simple Carbohydrate	
	Fat/oil	

Chocolate Milk

Eating	Protein	
	Complex carbohydrate	
	Simple Carbohydrate	
	Fat/oil	

Nuts

Eating	Protein	
	Complex carbohydrate	
	Simple Carbohydrate	
	Fat/oil	

Tuna salad sandwich

Eating	Protein	
	Complex carbohydrate	
	Simple Carbohydrate	
	Fat/oil	

Cheese and crackers

Eating	Protein		
	Complex carbohydrate		
	Simple Carbohydrate		
	Fat/oil		

Vegetables and dip

Eating	Protein		
	Complex carbohydrate		
	Simple Carbohydrate		
	Fat/oil		

Buttered Popcorn

Eating	Protein		
	Complex carbohydrate		
	Simple Carbohydrate		
	Fat/oil		

Fried Mexican Food

Eating	Protein		
	Complex carbohydrate		
	Simple Carbohydrate		
	Fat/oil		

Candy

Eating	Protein		
	Complex carbohydrate		
	Simple Carbohydrate		
	Fat/oil		

Cookies

Eating	Protein		
	Complex carbohydrate		
	Simple Carbohydrate		
	Fat/oil		

Ice cream

Eating	Protein	
	Complex carbohydrate	
	Simple Carbohydrate	
	Fat/oil	

French Fries

Eating	Protein	
	Complex carbohydrate	
	Simple Carbohydrate	
	Fat/oil	

Here's how I rated each item:

Buttered potatoes

Eating	Protein	
	Complex carbohydrate	•S
	Simple Carbohydrate	
	Fat/oil	•

Fried chicken

Eating	Protein	•
	Complex carbohydrate	
	Simple Carbohydrate	•
	Fat/oil	•

Salad with dressing

Eating	Protein	
	Complex carbohydrate	•V
	Simple Carbohydrate	
	Fat/oil	•

Chocolate Milk

Eating	Protein	•
	Complex carbohydrate	
	Simple Carbohydrate	•
	Fat/oil	

Nuts

Eating	Protein	•
	Complex carbohydrate	
	Simple Carbohydrate	
	Fat/oil	

Tuna salad sandwich

Eating	Protein	•
	Complex carbohydrate	
	Simple Carbohydrate	•
	Fat/oil	•

Cheese and crackers

Eating	Protein	•
	Complex carbohydrate	
	Simple Carbohydrate	•
	Fat/oil	

Notice I didn't put an S in the simple carb box. There's no need. All simple carbs are either sugar or starch.

Vegetables and dip

Eating	Protein	
	Complex carbohydrate	•V
	Simple Carbohydrate	
	Fat/oil	•

Candy

Eating	Protein	
	Complex carbohydrate	
	Simple Carbohydrate	•
	Fat/oil	

Cookies

Eating	Protein	
	Complex carbohydrate	
	Simple Carbohydrate	•
	Fat/oil	•

Ice cream

Eating	Protein	
	Complex carbohydrate	
	Simple Carbohydrate	•
	Fat/oil	•

Note that ice cream does not get a protein credit. The appetite switch isn't paying any attention to the protein aspect of ice cream.

Buttered Popcorn

Eating	Protein	
	Complex carbohydrate	•S
	Simple Carbohydrate	
	Fat/oil	•

Corn chips

Eating	Protein	
	Complex carbohydrate	
	Simple Carbohydrate	•
	Fat/oil	•

French Fries

Eating	Protein	
	Complex carbohydrate	
	Simple Carbohydrate	•
	Fat/oil	•

You may wonder why the corn chips and French fries aren't getting credit as complex carbs. After all, many Mexican wraps are made from corn.

Complex carbs, when they are starchy and fried, affect the appetite switch just as if they were simple carbs. All fried starches get recorded as simple carbs (and fat).

Day 3 Tools

Tomorrow, each time you eat, you will place a dot in the appropriate food categories that comprise your meal. By recording your food intake this way, you'll accomplish two things.

✧ You'll have a record of your eating without writing everything down.

✧ You'll be training yourself to see your food as chemicals.

Here are some examples:

Fried chicken, mashed potatoes, green beans, cookies, and milk

Eating	Protein	•
	Complex carbohydrate	•
	Simple Carbohydrate	•
	Fat/oil	•

Hamburger, fries, Dr. Pepper

Eating	Protein	•
	Complex carbohydrate	
	Simple Carbohydrate	•
	Fat/oil	•

Pasta, red sauce, salad and dressing, garlic bread, wine

Eating	Protein	•
	Complex carbohydrate	•
	Simple Carbohydrate	•
	Fat/oil	•

Vegetable soup

Eating	Protein	
	Complex carbohydrate	• V
	Simple Carbohydrate	
	Fat/oil	

Clam chowder

Eating	Protein	•
	Complex carbohydrate	•
	Simple Carbohydrate	•
	Fat/oil	•

Salmon, roasted potatoes, salad, dressing, asparagus

Eating	Protein	•
	Complex carbohydrate	•
	Simple Carbohydrate	
	Fat/oil	•

Today's To-Do List

1. Copy any of the Day 3 tools you want to take with you tomorrow.

2. Put your Training Week Chart, Day 3 beside your bed so you'll be ready to start charting as soon as you awaken.

3. Remember that you are learning a new way of looking at what you eat, so cut yourself some slack. Allow for a learning curve. Before long you'll be rating your meals very quickly.

FAQ

Q Why do you put some complex carbs into the simple carb category. I'm an expert on food composition and I know that juice, canned fruit, and dried fruit are complex carbs, and so is multigrain bread.

A I'm attending to the way each food affects the appetite switch in the brain, rather than presenting a strict analysis of the food itself. Fruit, when it's juiced, dried, or canned with syrup, becomes such a concentrated sweet that it affects the brain almost as if it were table sugar. Raisins are the exception because—drum roll—they are small. If you have no more than 10 raisins, that can count as a complex carb.

The same deal exists with multigrain bread, crackers, and cereals. Only if they are a 100% whole grain, can they be counted as a complex carb.

Fried foods, such as fried chicken or fish, get counted as a protein and as a fat and a simple carb. Anything that's breaded also gets a dot in the simple carb category.

Milk is a drink, but it's counted as a food—protein.

We'll get into more complex combos soon, but for now you have enough on your plate.

Food Chart

Food Type	Protein	Comp. Carb	Simp. Carb	Fat
Meat, fish	•			
Fried meat	•			•
Fried breaded meat or fish	•		•	•

Food Type	Protein	Comp. Carb	Simp. Carb	Fat
Veggie		•V		
Fried non-starch veggie		•V		•
Fried, breaded, non-starch veg.		•V	•	•
Beans (Navy, chili, red, black, etc.)		• S		
Most breads & cereals			•	
Rice (white)			•	
Potato		• S		
Oatmeal		• S		
Popcorn		• S		
Whole grain breads, rice, cereals		• S		
Fruit		• F		
Fruit-canned or dried			•	
Fried starch			•	•
Sugar/candy			•	
Most desserts			•	•
Peanut butter (all nuts)	•			
Peanut butter (w sugar & shortening)			•	•
Ice cream			•	•
Alcohol, wine, beer, etc			•	

Data Chart, Day 3

Basic Data--Training Week, Day 3		Time of Day	5	6	7	8	9	10	11	12	1	2	3	4	5	6	7	8	9	10	11	12	1	2	3	4
		Circle Wake-up Time																								
Appetite	Can't stop																										
	More food																										
	Craving food																										
	Food focused																										
	Quiet																										
Hunger	Starved																										
	Strong																										
	Moderate																										
	Mild																										
	Not hungry																										
Eating	Protein																										
	Comp carb																										
	Simp carb																										
	Fat/oil																										

8 Day 3

Today

Today, you are learning to work with a new system for recording food chemicals that enter your body. It doesn't have to be done perfectly. You do not have to be exacting. You do not have to google the food values of each food you eat.

1. Carry your chart with you today, and pause each hour to assess and mark your degrees of hunger and appetite.//
2. Whenever you eat anything, dot the categories that apply to the chemicals in your food.
3. At the end of the day, connect the dots in the hunger and appetite sections.

Jules' Third Day

If it would help, you can see how Jules marked her food chart. Jules had oatmeal for breakfast. She added some walnuts to it.

Here's how she marked her chart.

Basic Data--Training Week		Circle Wake-up Time						
		Time of Day	5	6	7	8	9	10
Eating	Protein					•		
	Complex carbohydrate						•S	
	Simple Carbohydrate							
	Fat/oil							

Oatmeal is a complex carb. Nuts are protein.

For lunch, Jules had a hamburger with lettuce, onion, and tomato, and a side salad with thousand island dressing.

Basic Data--Training Week		Circle Wake-up Time												
		Time of Day	5	6	7	8	9	10	11	12	1	2	3	4
Eating	Protein					•				•		•		
	Comp carb				•S					•V			V	
	Simple Carb									•				
	Fat/oil									•				

At 3:00 PM, Jules had some celery and cheese.

For dinner she had a sausage and pepperoni pizza and a beer. Sausage is a mixed food. It is composed of both fat and protein. All mixed foods are rated according to their most plentiful component. For example, bacon, sausage, and peanut butter are all more fat than protein, so they are treated as fats (unless the peanut butter is made entirely from nuts).

All alcohol is made from either sugar or starch, so it is treated as a simple carb.

After dinner, she couldn't stop eating and had a series of sugar and fat foods. Here's how her eating chart looked for the day:

Basic Data--Training Week		Circle Wake-up Time																		
		Time of Day	5	6	⑦	8	9	10	11	12	1	2	3	4	5	6	7	8	9	10 11
Eating	Protein					•				•		•								
	Comp carb				•S					•V			V							
	Simple Carb									•							•	•	•	•
	Fat/oil									•								•	•	•

FAQ

Q Do tacos or tostadas get a different rating than burritos?

A Fried corn or wheat products get treated the same as French fries. Even if they are from 100% whole grain, frying them turns them into an appetite trigger. Any starch that is fried is rated as a simple carb.

Here's a way to test this. When you have a nacho, potato chip, or French fry, do you eat one and then lose interest in having any more? Can you set a limit for yourself, such as 3 and stop there if the basket still has more nachos in it? If you continue to nibble, even if there are pauses between nibbles, that's a sign your appetite switch is being activated.

And what happens with baked potato chips? I'm betting after a small handful, chewing them is not worth the effort. So compare the intensity of your involvement with baked chips versus fried chips. That's the difference between a food that has no charge for the appetite switch, and one that activates it.

Q If I have nachos before my bean burrito and rice, how should I figure my meal. The nachos are fried, but the burrito wrap is not.

A Because nachos are fried, they are counted as a simple carb. The rice and wrap on the burrito are both simple carbs. The beans are a complex carb and also a starch. This is a meal high in starch. It would be rated as follows:

Protein	
Complex carbs	•S
Simple carbs	•
Fats/oils	•

Q I thought rice and beans together created a protein. Why don't they get counted as such?

A It is true that certain combinations of food provide enough complementary amino acids to produce a complete protein that can then be used as a building block in the body. But on the way to that happy outcome, these foods are still starches and have the power, in quantity, to trigger the appetite switch.

Q In the previous meal, can I count the lettuce and tomato garnish as a complex carb?

A Are you talking about a few shreds of lettuce and a sprinkle of small tomato wedges? And are you going to eat them or look at them? If there's enough lettuce and tomato to qualify as a small salad, (and you eat it rather than leave it on the plate), complex carbs do get a dot and a V. But if it's just a garnish, forggeddabout it.

Q My boss has a dish of candy in her office. When I'm in there, I pop a couple in my mouth. Can I forgeddabout it?

> **If you leave the vegetables on the plate and do not eat them, they don't get counted.**

A No. That's a simple carb and it gets counted, even if it's the only thing you eat that hour.

Q Are you saying I have to count one piece of candy?

A Yes. Remember your goal here. And remember that this isn't a diet. You are collecting data so that we can figure out what food chemicals are causing you to have a stuck appetite switch. The more honest you are about the foods that can affect the appetite switch, the more we will learn when we start testing your appetite chemicals, and the more effective your personal plan will be.

   I promise you this: you will not have to let go of any foods for at least a month and probably longer. And you'll decide what and when.

(But look at us, we're arguing. If we're in a fight about whether or not to count one piece of candy, that tells me that candy is really important. After all, we wouldn't be having this fight if it were a single green bean.

If you feel like defending candy when you wouldn't give a bean the time of day, it's a good sign that candy is having a very special effect on your brain. We'll talk about this later.)

Q If all I have is a pat of butter, do I have to put a dot in the fats box?
A Yes. If all you have in one hour is a pat of butter, put a dot in the fats box.

Q So I have to count one piece of candy, but not a small vegetable garnish.
A True. Remember that the lettuce garnish was on a big burrito with beans, rice, and fried corn chips. Those few fibers got totally swamped by the starch in the meal.
Notice you're starting to think a 4 letter word--*diet*. Wanting to quibble about whether or not a food counts (wanting to 'be good') is at the fringes of the diet mentality. Back away from that. You're turning off your appetite switch. Remember?

Q Doesn't quantity matter?
A It does and it doesn't. For our purposes here—for gathering basic data about what is causing you to have a stuck appetite switch—we don't need to look at ounces, calories, or units in order to see what's happening with your appetite switch. We can tell a lot just by seeing if the dots are mostly at the bottom of the chart.

Quantity does matter when the additive effect of various components of your meal mean that you are deluging your brain with carbs. A load of starchy carbs, even if complex, can affect your appetite switch, and if it does, we need a record of it. We need to see what that kind of meal does to your appetite and hunger values over the course of a day.

Example: High starch meal despite the presence of complex carbohydrates.

Protein	
Complex carbs	•S
Simple carbs	•
Fats/oils	•

9 Getting Ready for Day 4

Preparing for Tomorrow, Day 4

We'll make tomorrow an easy one since you're still scratching your head over how to rate your meals. Tomorrow you'll just make one more discrimination regarding your intake. If any food or drink you eat has caffeine in it, you'll check a box at the bottom of the food section.

Research Tool 4—Caffeine Intake

If you have coffee, tea, or chocolate, you'll check the caffeine box for that hour.

Tomorrow you'll find one other item on your chart. You'll notate whether or not you had any problems with sleep tonight—either trouble getting to sleep, restless sleep, or waking up and not returning to sleep very easily.

By the way, I have help for you if you want it. Go to my web site: www.master**your**appetite.com. Have this book with you. Enter a secret word that's in this book to get access to additional tools. You can also download your charts from there.

Later on we'll talk about food choices that affect a surprising array of non-eating issues. For example, one of the chemicals in your brain that affects your appetite also affects your willingness to exercise. When you restore this chemical, you'll get more interested in moving your body.

Another body chemical affects how vulnerable you feel. When you're a quart low of this biochemical, you are much more easily stressed and more raw and sensitive to the slights or meanness of others. When you rebuild this handy little chemical, not only will you become more bullet proof, it will also reduce hunger and appetite. So for the bargain price of one food, you get stress relief, hunger reduction, and a peaceful appetite. What a deal!

Stay tuned for these revelations. For now, we're just planning ahead by gathering data that you'll use later to see what a difference you are making for yourself.

By the way, if you drink something with sugar in it, be sure to count that in your simple carb row.

Today's To-Do List

1. Make a copy of the Training Week, Day 4 chart unless you are going to write in your book.

2. Put that chart next to your bed so it will be there for you to make your first mark in the morning.

3. When you wake up tomorrow, circle the time you wake up, and then mark your hunger and appetite ratings. If you had problems with your sleep, mark that also.

Data Chart 4

Basic Data--Training Week, Day 4		Circle Wake-up Time																						
	Time of Day	5	6	7	8	9	10	11	12	**1**	**2**	**3**	**4**	**5**	**6**	**7**	**8**	**9**	10	11	12	1	2	3	4
Appetite	Can't stop																								
	More food																								
	Craving food																								
	Food focused																								
	Quiet																								
Hunger	Starved																								
	Strong																								
	Moderate																								
	Mild																								
	Not hungry																								
Eating	Protein																								
	Comp carb																								
	Simp carb																								
	Fat/oil																								
Caffeine	Yes																								
Mark the following items just once each day. You can use a mark or make a note for your answer.																									
Sleep Problems																									

FAQ

Q It's hard for me to think of being completely honest about what I'm eating, even to myself.

A Yes, if you're like most of us, you've been fudging about what you're actually eating. We tend to slice off bits of the truth when we report our food to anyone (or to ourselves).

We've had so many years of feeling guilty about eating that we may feel guilt or shame no matter what we eat, even if it's healthy. All the time I hear women apologize for eating, as if we aren't supposed to need food.

Even though no one will see your charts except you, that guilt may be aroused just by noticing that you are eating. That's why I want you to pause and really absorb the fact that you've been forced to eat. The appetite switch in your brain has made you eat whether you wanted to or not.

Every time you dieted, you were trying to defy your appetite switch. But it is stronger than you are and it beat you, right? Even Oprah, with all her helpers and all her determination, has had that appetite switch take hold of her at times and drag her back into old eating. The appetite switch always wins in the long run.

Your best hope is to fix your appetite switch. And over time, your eating will change, automatically. This is not a quick fix, even though you'll be able to notice some changes within a month. But it is a **reliable** fix. So settle down, find some patience, and remember what you're doing just for today.

Q Why aren't you having me record my beverages? Any other diet book tells me to drink 8 glasses of water a day.

A First, this isn't a diet book. It's a change-your-brain book.

Second, didn't you already get told to drink 8 glasses of water a day? And are you doing it?

Since you already know being flushed is good for you, you don't need that from me. Besides, if you generally deprive your body of what it needs, then not drinking water may be a part of that pattern.

I'm confident that two things will happen. First, you'll start to exercise spontaneously after your chemicals re-balance, and exercise always forces us to drink more fluid. Second, when you start to like your body more—once you prove to yourself that it hasn't been mean to you when it made you eat—you'll be nicer to it.

Third, as your stress level drops when you learn the tricks I'm going to teach you, you'll start to have more common sense (not that sense is common). So you'll realize that a tendency to eat or drink whatever is in front of you can be used to your advantage. You'll get one of those giant water bottles, fill it in the morning, drag it with you wherever you go, and your own compulsion will cause you to drink it down.

Q. Are you serious? Do I have to rate what's in my drinks?

A. Yes. You are to include any intake that has food value whether it comes in the form of a liquid or a solid. It doesn't matter if it's a food or a beverage. Sugar gets counted even in a liquid, as does the protein in milk, the fat in a hot buttered rum, the sugar in hot chocolate, the vegetables or starches in soup, or the simple carbs in any alcoholic beverage or soft drink.

You are mere days away from fixing your appetite switch

10 Training Week, Day 4

1. Mark your chart as soon as you wake up. Check your hunger and appetite ratings and indicate any problems you had falling or staying asleep last night.
2. Carry your chart with you today. Mark appetite and hunger levels each hour and the components of any food you eat, including caffeine.

Athlete Envy

Samantha felt very bad about herself. Every time she went to her doctor, he told her to exercise. She knew she should and often she promised him she would, but then when she got back into her real world, she didn't follow through.

Her friend, Lorna, was a faithful runner. She got up every morning and ran a loop around their neighborhood. Samantha envied Lorna's discipline and would compare herself to Lorna, feeling like an inferior being because she couldn't manage a similar program.

One of her friends, Tayler, was the sort who always knew how everyone else should run their lives. Tay would tell her, "Samantha, just start. Set a time every day, and just walk from your house to the bus stop.

Start with that. Then add a block a week."

It sounded reasonable, but still, Samantha never ended up finding the time. She'd gotten to the point where she agreed with people's good suggestions, at the same time feeling bad from knowing she wouldn't be able to put any of them into action, no matter how simple they seemed. And she resented it too, that everyone had such easy advice and had no understanding about how something in her just wouldn't let her exercise. It was a big immovable block she couldn't get past.

When she started this program, she expected me to tell her to exercise, and when I didn't, she brought it up. "Why aren't you telling me to exercise. It's like a sword hanging over my head, waiting for you to push me."

I told her, "I don't have to tell you to exercise. When your appetite switch gets better, you'll starting moving on your own."

She made a sound like air squeezed out of a bicycle tire and said, "Yeah, when it snows in Hell."

A few months later, she told her group. "I joined a gym today." She said it casually, like, "I got the mail today."

Her group was delighted for her and very supportive. Not one of them gasped or fainted.

I said, "New weather report just in from Hell. It's snowing."

If you have a story like Samantha's, you've been blaming yourself for something your brain wouldn't let you do. When your appetite switch is out of whack, it can make you resistant to exercise.

You may have noticed that whatever exercise you manage to do, you have to force yourself to do it. Let's look at that now.

Your Relationship with Exercise and Food

Read each belief or action and mark *yes* if it is true.

Beliefs/Actions	Yes
1. I think I should exercise.	
2. I know my level of exercise is way below the recommended level for my age group.	
3. I hate exercise and can't make myself do it.	
4. I feel bad about not exercising enough.	
5. I have to force myself to exercise.	
6. I think I should make better food choices.	
7. I know my nutritional choices are below recommended standards.	
8. I know I eat more than is good for me.	
9. I know my eating is not in a healthy balance.	
10. I can't sustain healthier eating for as long as I'd like.	
11. I have to force myself to eat in a healthier way.	
Totals	

What did you discover?

Questions 1 and 6 are belief questions. They indicate what you think you *should* be doing. The other questions give information about how your actions are matching your beliefs. The more *yes* answers you have in the unshaded rows, the more certain it is that your appetite switch is controlling your food and exercise choices.

Force

Questions 5 and 11 are the force questions. Two *yes* answers here indicate that you are forcing yourself too much. Force causes stress, rebellion, and growing resistance. These backfire eventually.

Are you noticing just how much force you use to make yourself do what you think you should? Force doesn't last, does it? You can only force yourself to do something for so long and then you simply can't keep pushing yourself to continue.

How would you like to be able to exercise and eat differently without resorting to force? How would it be to look forward to exercise?

What if eating more healthfully required only a modicum of discipline now and then? What if exercising took only a mild push part of the time?

Since both of these factors are controlled by the appetite switch, you can reach this happy state. Your appetite switch determines whether or not you want to exercise. It also controls your food choices and your portion size.

By fixing your appetite switch, you will add movement to your life spontaneously, not using any force at all. Imagine that?

Imagine, you'll want to exercise.

Preparing for Tomorrow, Day 5

Tomorrow you'll start noticing whether you have a genuine desire to exercise. It's one more piece of baseline data. Later, when you start some sort of movement spontaneously, you'll be able to look back and appreciate how much you've done for yourself by fixing your appetite switch.

Tomorrow's chart will include a brief form of the yes or no question, "Did you genuinely feel like exercising today?" Answer honestly, and when the day comes that you change your "no" answer to "yes," notice how long it took from now to then.

If you're interested, go to my website, www.annekatherine.org, and fill in the chart that asks how long it took. That will be an inspiration to others who can't believe they'd ever *want* to exercise.

Today's Tasks

1. Make a copy of the Training Week, Day 5 chart unless you are going to carry this book with you and use the chart in the book.
2. Put that chart (or this book) next to your bed so it will be there for you to make your first mark in the morning.
3. When you wake up tomorrow, circle the time you wake up, and then mark your hunger and appetite ratings. If you had problems with your sleep, mark that also.

Basic Data--Training Week, Day 5		Circle Wake-up Time	
	Time of Day	5 6 7 8 9 10 11 12 **1 2 3 4 5 6 7 8 9** 10 11 12 1 2 3 4	
Appetite	Can't stop		
	More food		
	Craving food		
	Food focused		
	Quiet		
Hunger	Starved		
	Strong		
	Moderate		
	Mild		
	Not hungry		
Eating	Protein		
	Comp carb		
	Simp carb		
	Fat/oil		
Caffeine	Yes		

Mark the following items just once each day. You can use a mark or make a note for your answer.				
Sleep Problems		Felt like exercising.	Yes	No

FAQ

Q Don't you just *have* to make yourself do some things? Isn't that realistic?

A Are you looking for an all or none answer here? Do I do things everyday that I don't enjoy? Yes, of course. I don't like to floss, but I do it. Do I force myself? No, because I established a routine and the routine carries me through.

If you have compulsive tendencies like most of us who compulsively eat, you can use that to your advantage. Knowing I will drink whatever is in the glass in front of me, I fill a really large glass with slightly flavored water and put it beside my computer. Then while I'm working compulsively, I automatically drink my water and get my fluids for the day.

Knowing my hands like to be busy (and that I think flossing in the bathroom is boring), I put my dental floss on a little shelf next to where I watch TV. In the evening, my hands find that floss and my teeth get taken care of.

Gaining access to this way of working with yourself is one of the resources that will become available to you as you decrease your hours of self-blame, shame, guilt, and force. You can turn what seem like faults to your advantage when you begin to shift your self-perspective toward acceptance and away from finger-shaking.

You've been blaming yourself for what your brain has been directing. Your vital research this week will make this very clear when you take the first test and notice how your data changes as a result.

The baseline data that you are compiling this week will affect your brain in and of itself—by changing what you believe about yourself as you see that your eating improves ever more as you fix your appetite switch.

You'll eat differently as your appetite switch gets fixed.

11   Training Week, Day 5

1. Mark your chart as soon as you wake up. Check your hunger and appetite ratings and indicate any problems you had falling or staying asleep last night.
2. Carry your chart with you today and mark appetite and hunger levels each hour, and the components of any food you eat, including caffeine.
3. Tonight, after you connect the dots, look back over the day to see if you felt like exercising. Notice, you aren't recording any exercise, only if you *felt* like exercising. Mark *yes* if you genuinely wanted to exercise. Mark *no* if you thought you should exercise, forced yourself to exercise, or felt guilty for not exercising.

Preparing for tomorrow, Day 6

Today we'll consider a new word—satiety. Satiety means you have enough of something. You are satisfied, complete, sated. With regard to eating, satiety means that your appetite has been satisfied.

Although satiety has a popular definition as just noted, when it relates to your brain chemistry, it refers to a physiological state—one in which the body stops pushing for something because it is chemically complete.

Satiety biochemicals stop appetite chemicals. For overeaters, these are the good guys. We want them. We want to build them up and support them.

For the next three weeks you are going to take specific actions that will increase your satiety body chemicals, so tomorrow, you will start noticing when you have reached satiety. This adds to the research you've already been doing and gives us additional baseline information.

Today you might begin to pay attention to your body and notice when it feels satisfied. If you're like many of us who have binge eating disorder, you may have never felt satisfied. Most of the women I've worked with just looked at me cross-eyed when I started talking about having enough. They'd stopped eating because someone came home, the bag was empty, or they'd fallen into a stupor, but hardly ever because they'd felt completely satisfied.

Research Tool 6—Satiety

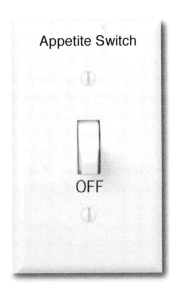

Tomorrow, when you pause to consider your hunger and appetite levels, you'll also notice whether or not you are pulled toward food or eating. If you are, put a dot in the "not satisfied" row. That means you *don't* have satiety.

If you are *not* pulled toward food or eating, put a dot in the "satisfied" row. That means you have satiety.

Basic Data--Training Week, Day 6		Circle Wake-up Time																				
	Time of Day	5	6	7	8	9	10	11	12	1	2	3	4	5	6	7	8	9	10	11	12	1	2	3	4
Appetite	Can't stop																						
	More food																						
	Craving food																						
	Food focused																						
	Quiet																						
Hunger	Starved																						
	Strong																						
	Moderate																						
	Mild																						
	Not hungry																						
Eating	Protein																						
	Comp carb																						
	Simp carb																						
	Fat/oil																						
Caffeine	Yes																						
Satiety	Not satisfied																						
	Satisfied																						

llowing items just once each day. You can use a mark or make a note for y

Sleep Problems		Felt like exercising.	Yes	No	

FAQ

Q I'm confused. I'm supposed to mark *Satisfied* if I'm *not* pulled to eating and *Not satisfied* if I *am* pulled to eating.

A You can think of it like this:

- ✧ If you are pulled toward food or eating in this moment, mark the box in the top shaded row.
- ✧ If you are not being drawn toward food or eating for the moment, mark the box in the bottom shaded row.

Q I don't know what you are talking about. I have no concept of satiety.

A Join the club. You are among thousands of other adults who also don't relate to this idea. I wouldn't normally ask you to do something that is so foreign, but the value of looking inside and getting curious about what satiety feels like is this—one day you will realize that you have absolutely no interest in eating, and this will be a very exciting moment.

This will tell you two things:
- ✧ That your satiety chemicals have started working
- ✧ What normal people feel like.

Who knew? The reason normal people don't overeat? They lose interest in food. It's just that easy. It's not (in most cases) from will power or being a superior person or having mega-doses of self-control. It's from having a full tank of satiety chemicals.

You will be learning how to fill your tank.

You'll look normal too. (Don't worry. You'll still be the interesting, creative, wonderful person you are now.)

12 Day 6

Today's To-do List

1. Follow your usual protocol.
2. Notice whether or not you are drawn to food or eating. If you are not pulled to food or eating, mark the bottom shaded row in the *Satiety* category. If food is calling you, mark the top shaded row.

Stress

We just have one more thing to track and then you're good to go. Tomorrow you're going to rate your stress level. Stress is an important process to track because it stimulates comfort eating.

You've probably heard of eating for comfort. Some of us (like about 90 million[3]) turn to food in order to soothe ourselves.

Why does that work? Why would food be soothing? Plus, some food is, some isn't. Why isn't all food soothing?

I love broccoli, but that's not what I want when six things go wrong and some jerk waves a finger at me as he crowds me off the road. No,

---

[3] Based on the possibility that only half of overweight Americans overeat in order to soothe themselves.

broccoli is a very nice vegetable, but it is of little help if I want to be rocked like a baby.

These questions will be answered, but for now, we just want to start measuring how stressful your life is.

Two reasons:

1. A deficiency of a brain chemical makes stress more stressful.
2. We want to see if you are more easily soothed when we start fixing your brain.

All her life, Talia had suffered from her family's ridicule over being what they saw as hyper-sensitive. Touchy Talia they called her, even after she was married and a successful realtor.

She did seem to notice rudeness other people brushed off. A mean comment from their uncle would feel like a claw in her gut whereas her sister merely called him a drunk and went about her business. Many a night she fretted or worried over a chance comment from her boss, while her husband's perspective was that Talia was their best agent and the broker would be crazy to lose her.

Talia had unwritten lists of rules that she followed to prevent people from being upset with her. She tried to do everything perfectly. She'd go more than the extra mile with her clients, like about an extra ten miles. She worked way past the time fatigue made her legs heavy. If everyone else brought one dish to a potluck, she'd bring an extra side and a vase of flowers. Her to-do list was longer than anyone could possibly accomplish in a single day, and she drove herself to complete as many items as she could. Then she'd feel bad about the items she couldn't cross off.

The way she stopped this incessant pressure was by eating and watching TV. At the end of the day she ate non-stop while watching television, and this put the press-gang to sleep.

She never dreamed her lack of insulation was caused by a scarce brain chemical. After a couple of months on this program, she noticed that she wasn't so concerned about her boss's approval. She wasn't walking around like a satellite dish picking up every mean comment in her vicinity. What a relief.

As her attention moved from her outsides to her insides, she became aware that she actually wanted to work for a different company, and she had the strength to make the switch, despite her broker's reaction.

Just a little chemical made a huge difference.

Tomorrow's research will help show if your anti-stress chemical is working properly. First you'll record how stressed you are now before you activate the anti-stress chemical, and later what happens after you activate it.

Here's the chart you'll use tomorrow:

Basic Data--Training Week, Day 7		Circle Wake-up Time																						
	Time of Day	5	6	7	8	9	10	11	12	**1**	**2**	**3**	**4**	**5**	**6**	**7**	**8**	**9**	10	11	12	1	2	3	4
Appetite	Can't stop																								
	More food																								
	Craving food																								
	Food focused																								
	Quiet																								
Hunger	Starved																								
	Strong																								
	Moderate																								
	Mild																								
	Not hungry																								
Eating	Protein																								
	Comp carb																								
	Simp carb																								
	Fat/oil																								
Caffeine	Yes																								
Satiety	Not satisfied																								
	Satisfied																								
Sress	High																								
	Medium																								
	Low																								
	None																								

Mark the following items just once each day. You can use a mark or make a note for your answer.

Sleep Problems		Felt like exercising.	Yes	No	

Today's Tasks—Preparing for tomorrow

1. Make a copy of the Training Week, Day 7 chart unless you are going to carry this book with you and use the chart in the book.
2. Put that chart (or this book) next to your bed so it will be there for you to make your first mark in the morning.
3. When you wake up tomorrow, circle the time you wake up, and then mark your hunger and appetite ratings.
4. Then notice whether or not food is calling you. If not, mark the bottom shaded row in the *Satiety* category. If so, mark the top shaded row.
5. Next, notice your stress level. Put a dot in either the "None," "Low," "Medium," or "High" box.
6. If you had problems with your sleep, mark that also.

FAQ

Q Tonight, do I connect all the dots, even in the satiety row?

A Yes, connect the dots horizontally across each individual category as shown below. Tomorrow night, you'll even connect the dots across the stress rows. The only dots that don't get connected are those in the Eating subcategories. See the example below.

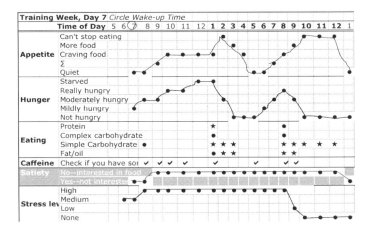

13 Training Week, Last Day

Congratulations

Look at what you've accomplished in one week.

- ✧ You've learned to use 7 research tools so you can test the major biochemicals that affect your appetite switch.
- ✧ You've collected the data you will compare to the results of those tests.
- ✧ You've learned some techniques you can use to slow yourself down and to give yourself more choices.

You are one week into creating the habit of a daily protocol that will help you stay conscious about your best goals for yourself.

If you got here legitimately, by reading each chapter in order and taking a couple of small steps each day, this protocol should start getting easier. Since you added just one new tool each day, you gave yourself your best shot at keeping the overwhelm at a manageable level.

Congratulations once again. You were extraordinarily good to yourself.

> **If you jumped here and didn't follow the Training Week chapters day-by-day, take a look at this.**
>
> **Is this your pattern? Does it cause you to miss bits of info that other people seem to have? Does it set you up to be so overwhelmed that you abandon the direction you were heading? Does it defeat you and keep you from reaching your goals?**
>
> **If any of this is familiar, think about whether you want to challenge this costly pattern of yours. Are you curious about what it would be like to try a different pattern? If so, go back to the beginning and come back through the Training Week days one-by-one.**
>
> **Honestly, you really do have a tool here that can make your life much more manageable. Give it an honest shot at working.**

This is the last day you'll be collecting basic data. Tomorrow you'll start the first test on your brain. The protocol that we've been building step-by-step will be your modus operandi for 3 more weeks. You will use this

Daily Protocol

1. Mark your chart as soon as you awaken.
2. You know how to mark each category.
3. Carry your chart with you throughout the day and pause hourly to check your appetite, hunger, stress, and satiety levels.
4. Record the components of any food you eat.
5. Connect the dots at the end of the day and answer any remaining questions on your chart.

same protocol to collect data as you give yourself each test.

Each week you will test your appetite switch by making one change. You'll use a special data chart for each week. At the end of each week, you'll have data on how that test affected your appetite switch.

Taken together, the first three tests will show you that you can considerably lower the amps on your appetite switch, and you will automatically begin eating smaller meals, have more energy, and be less stressed.

Test 1.

Tomorrow you'll begin the first test by changing one thing about your eating. If it lowers your appetite switch, you'll have discovered that the chemical NPY is making you eat.

Here's the test. Eat every two to three hours. Add two snacks to your three daily meals.

The meals can be anything you want, as long as they have some protein. **The snacks can be anything *but* wheat, sugar, flour, artificial sweetener, or simple carbs. Snacks must not have a flavor enhancer like msg. Stevia and xylitol are the only acceptable alternative sweeteners** for snacks.

You don't have to change anything else about your eating. You don't have to add any particular foods. You don't have to subtract any particular foods. You do have to rearrange your eating.

FAQ

Q I don't eat breakfast.

A Then you have an opportunity to do some real good for yourself.

Skipping breakfast sets up a drastic NPY response later in the day. If you routinely skip breakfast or any other meals, make some room for a learning curve. Besides adding two snacks a day, you'll also be adding breakfast or any other skipped meals. Thus you'll be making two changes. You might want to take two weeks to do this—one week to add breakfast and another week to add two snacks.

Here are some examples:

Example 1.

Breakfast: Deviled egg on wheat toast, coffee with cream

Snack: soup (with no msg)

Lunch: hamburger and fries, salad, dessert

Snack: apple

Dinner: fried chicken, mashed potatoes and gravy, salad, roll and butter.

> **Test 1**
> 1. Eat every 2 or 3 hours.
> 2. To be counted as a legitimate meal, you must eat some protein.
> 3. To be counted as a legitimate snack, it must *not* have:
>   a. Wheat
>   b. Sugar
>   c. Flour
>   d. *Artificial* sweetener
>   e. Msg
>   f. Simple carbs

Example 2

B: cereal with banana and milk, tea, orange juice

S: V8 juice

L: Tomato soup, grilled cheese sandwich, pickles, cookies

S: Salad with dressing (no croutons)

D: Beef stew, salad with 1000 island dressing and croutons, biscuit, dessert

Example 3

B: Granola with raisins and milk, coffee with cream

S: Ham salad

L: Fish and chips, slaw, garlic bread

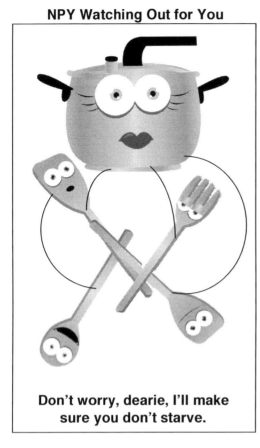

NPY Watching Out for You

Don't worry, dearie, I'll make sure you don't starve.

S: grapes

D: meat loaf, mashed potatoes, salad with ranch dressing, corn, bread and butter, ice cream

Timing

Breakfast should occur within one hour of awakening. All succeeding meals and snacks should occur within two to three hours of the previous meal or snack.

Test 1 will mellow your blood sugar.

Spikes and troughs in blood sugar and insulin create false hunger and uneven drops in energy. This causes extra eating and also slows your engine down at intervals, interrupting calorie burning and **causing the manufacture of fat**.

(Where do you think that sugar goes when insulin takes it out of your blood? It gets converted to fat. It goes straight to your thighs, or your bottom, or your…whatever.)

Test 1 will begin to lower your NPY level.

Neuropeptide Y is a potent appetite stimulator. It turns your appetite switch ON. I'm not talking a little bit on. I'm talking full out, voracious, bring me more food **ON**.

Whenever you delay or skip a meal, NPY begins to accumulate. It doesn't bother you while you're *not* eating. It bothers you a lot when you *start* eating later.

After skipping or delaying a meal, NPY silently gathers, waiting, waiting. It's smart. It figures, you don't have any food or you'd eat. So food must be scarce. OK. I'll just wait. I'll wait till you have food. Once you find a mammoth, microwave it, and start to eat, then I'll act. I'll make you eat a lot, so you're ready for the next famine.

NPY is a huge culprit when it comes to overeating. When it controls your appetite switch you absolutely can't overrule it. It is much stronger than you are—as much as 50 times stronger than other appetite stimulants—and it will *make* you eat. Please note, you cannot talk yourself out of NPY-influenced eating. It *will* control you.

How to Have a Choice

Never, ever skip or delay a meal or snack. Always eat something every two to three hours. Always, always—and I mean this—always eat breakfast.

You don't have to eat breakfast food. You just have to eat. You can have soup, salad, a sandwich, a drumstick, meat loaf. I don't care. But you must have some protein, and the cream in your coffee is not enough.

It doesn't have to be a big meal. You can have one hard-boiled egg or ten peanuts. Just have something within the first hour you get up.

How to Set Yourself Up to Binge

Skip breakfast.

Anytime, every time, you skip breakfast, whether it's tomorrow or four months from now, you will activate your NPY. It will accumulate throughout the morning and for as long as you delay eating.

Once you take your first bite sometime in the day, it will pounce on you. It will make you want more food and it will make your eating last much longer than if you'd had breakfast.

Are You NPY vulnerable?

To find out, take this test.

Question	Yes	No
Did you try your first diet when you were eighteen or younger?		
Have you tried more than 4 diets?		
Was even one of them extreme—as in very low calorie or liquid?		
Did you find it harder to stay on each successive diet?		
Were you less successful with each later diet?		
Have you lost faith in your ability to diet?		
Can you go all day without eating and not be bothered by it?		
After skipping a meal or two, do you get more food than you planned when you do start eating?		
After skipping a meal or two, do you continue eating after your next meal would normally be done? (Or does it not finish for a long time?)		
After skipping a meal or two, at your next meal, do you want more food even if you have to stop eating due to social pressure?		

If you answered yes to at least five questions, the odds are you are now NPY vulnerable. This means your NPY is easily activated, even by *delaying* a meal.

You are not alone. You have oodles of buddies. Lots of us accidentally made ourselves vulnerable to NPY when we were teenagers.

Notice the shaded blocks in the questionnaire. A *yes* in those five blocks is the typical profile of a person who accidentally activated her appetite switch by scaring her body into thinking she lived in a world where famine occurred regularly.

Obviously this is a plot generated by nature to keep humans on the planet. Wisely or not (in terms of the planet's wellbeing), human beings are protected from extinction by NPY. It protects us from variations in the food supply so that we can function when we aren't eating and it makes the most of the opportunity when food shows up.

Throughout history, famine has been a threat to survival. Rarely in history has too much food been a problem. So you are genetically protected against starvation and have minimal programmed protection against too much food.

NPY does two other things—its slows metabolism and it makes you disinterested in exercise.

Hmm, what would happen to a person whose appetite drove her to eat while her metabolism was dropping and she couldn't make herself exercise? Would she gain weight? Of course. She can't help but gain weight.

This combo is a size XXX waiting to happen. In fact a person will get obese quickly when this chemical situation is going on in her body.

Remember, this ensures survival. If food is scarce, it's smart to conserve energy by lowering metabolism (probably by causing a drop in thyroid stimulation or production) and preventing exercise.

Add one more factor: species survival requires fertile females. Prime time baby production occurs for humans in late adolescence. In other words, at the exact time teenagers think they should be going on an extreme diet, nature thinks they should be preparing for motherhood. Teenage girls, going on their first diet, get an all-out, save-the-species response from NPY. Their potential motherhood is much more important to nature than size four jeans. (It doesn't worry so much about fathers. Dudes can squeeze out that seed in the most dire circumstances.)

This sets the ball rolling. No diet will be as possible to follow as the first one. Diet three will be harder than diet two. Dieters will abandon their plans sooner and sooner. Not because they are weak, but because their NPY shot up the minute they started restricting food.

Fast forward twenty or thirty years and you've got a woman with extra weight, lower metabolism, resistance to exercise, no faith in her ability to eat the way she wants to, and NPY watching for the first sign of famine—as in a delayed meal or—horrors—a skipped meal.

For a chemical that causes so much trouble—in any country with lots of food in every direction—it's shockingly easy to fix.

Just don't skip a meal and eat every two to three hours—so that you have five meals or snacks a day.

Never **P**ass-up **Y**our-Vittles

Nourishment **P**revents **Y**ens (for too much food)

(I admit. These slogans are a stretch, but if they help make an impression, I can stand the humiliation.)

Remember, when you pass-up your vittles, NPY is a time bomb waiting to explode your appetite.

Preparing for Tomorrow

1. Make 7 copies of the chart at the end of the chapter. You will use a fresh copy of these charts every day for the next week.
2. Make 7 copies of the Planning Place tool if you want to use it.
3. Get a notebook or folder for your first seven Basic Data/Training Week charts. (These are golden. We'll use these charts in many ways to measure your progress. They will prove to you that your brain is responsive to your new practices and that, even if it takes awhile for your weight to show a difference, your brain is changing in the direction that makes greater health, wholesome eating, and weight loss possible.)
4. Shop for foods you can use as snacks. (Food lists and a planning tool are at the end of the chapter.)
5. Shop for foods you will eat at breakfast.
6. Get baggies so that you can stash food at work and in your car.
7. Set aside 10 minutes after you shop to prepare your snacks.
8. Is today a weekend day or a day off from work? Then after you read this chapter, but before you go shopping, look at Chapter 15, "Your First Weekend (After Training Week)."
9. Set aside an hour during your next weekend to organize your snacks for easy use.
10. Put one fresh copy of your Test 1 Data Chart next to your bed. When you awaken tomorrow, before you get out of bed, dot the appropriate boxes for your first hour.

Sample Meal Items

Breakfast	
Asparagus	Nuts
Cereal	Potatoes
Cheese	Quiche
Egg sandwich	Sandwich
Eggs	Soy milk
Fruit	Spinach
Granola	Tomatoes
Meat	Yogurt
Lunch or Dinner	
Any of the above	Salad
Burritos	Seafood
Fruit	Soup
Gyro	Tostada
Pasta and sauce	Tuna
Pizza	Vegetables
Snacks	
Cheese	Pickles (No sugar)
Eggs	Raisins (10)
Fruit	Salad
Granola (no sugar)	Seafood
Meat	Soup
Nuts	Soy products
Olives	Tuna
Peanut butter	Veggies

Test 1 Data Chart

This chart looks very like the Training Week, Day 7 Basic Chart. The difference is that there's now a slot for the date. Be sure to fill in the date each day so that you can put them in order when you look at the data.

Basic Data--Test 1												Circle Wake-up Time										Date			
	Time of Day	5	6	7	8	9	10	11	12	**1**	**2**	**3**	**4**	**5**	**6**	**7**	**8**	**9**	10	11	12	1	2	3	4
Appetite	Can't stop																								
	More food																								
	Craving food																								
	Food focused																								
	Quiet																								
Hunger	Starved																								
	Strong																								
	Moderate																								
	Mild																								
	Not hungry																								
Eating	Protein																								
	Comp carb																								
	Simp carb																								
	Fat/oil																								
Caffeine	Yes																								
Satiety	Not satisfied																								
	Satisfied																								
Sress	High																								
	Medium																								
	Low																								
	None																								

Mark the following items just once each day. You can use a mark or make a note for your answer.

Sleep Problems		Felt like exercising.	Yes	No	

Quick Portable Meals

Pancake sandwiches--Buckwheat pancakes with a pineapple slice or apple or pear or peach slice in the middle, or spread with ricotta or cream cheese

Yogurt with granola and fruit topping

Eggs scrambled with green onions and asparagus in pita pocket

Quiche—individual serving size in the freezer dept.

Egg sandwich

Handful of nuts and raisins

Bacon sandwich and milk

Egg sandwich

Scrambled egg, roasted tomato burrito

Hard-cooked egg

Burrito filled with scrambled egg, cheese, salsa, and sour cream

Potatoes with cheese on top

Meat loaf sandwich

Tuna sandwich

Salad

Soup

Chicken pieces, slaw, apple

Pork chop, slaw, raisins

Meat balls, dipping sauce, salad, orange

Walking salad: cored apple filled with peanut butter, nuts, raisins, and/or cream cheese

After Shopping

Organize tomorrow's snacks into baggies.

If you have to make a quick getaway in the morning, fix your breakfast combination tonight and put it in a travel container next to your snack bags.

Before Bed

Put your Test 1 Data Chart next to your bed, ready for morning.

Phew! This was a big day.

Planning Place—Optional Tool

You don't have to use this. It's here for you if you like to make lists.

Mealtime	Meal items	Shopping list
Breakfast		
Snack		
Lunch		
Snack		
Dinner		

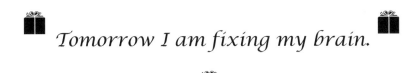

Tomorrow I am fixing my brain.

14   Week 1, Test 1

1. Follow your protocol.
2. Now, go eat breakfast before an hour passes.
3. Take your snacks with you today.

> **Did you get here legitimately by following the steps in the previous 7 chapters?**
>
> If so, you rock.
> If not, tsk, tsk.
> Go back, start reading at chapter 2, and get here by taking the 7 small steps that get you ready for this one.
> Really, this is no time to fight me. You can do that later when it will work to your advantage.

Overview

This chapter is only for those who've trained themselves to use the data charts correctly and who have taken the small daily steps to get themselves ready for today. Remember rule 1: **Take each change, each test, and each chapter in order.**

Good for you, you've exercised self control in the most effective way—by taking each chapter in order, learning your research tools, practicing those little steps that make possible big changes, and gathering the basic data that we'll use over and over to diagnose the problems with your appetite switch.

The Plan

The eating change you are making today will be the first test that will help in diagnosing the problem. **You will make this change and only this one change this week.** At the end of the week you can begin comparing the data from your charts this week to your basic data charts from last week.

Next week you'll give your brain a different test, and then look at the data from that week. Each week, after you test your brain, you will notice if your data changes. Any time your data improves after a week's testing, you'll know that you corrected a cause of your stuck appetite switch.

Eventually you'll have a profile that will tell you exactly what you have to do to keep your appetite switch turned off. As long as you follow that profile, your appetite will bother you less as time goes on.

Are you with me? If the previous paragraphs didn't make sense, don't worry. That's just the overview. We'll be taking it step-by-step and you'll catch on.

Rule 2

Make this one change and only this change this week.

This first test will tell us if NPY is making you eat. If so, it's easy to fix. If not, we'll know it doesn't have to be in your personal eating plan.

Don't add any other changes to your five meals or snacks a day. Don't start thinking you should only eat baked chicken and broiled fish. Don't let your mind trick you into thinking you should be dieting.

Remember, this is not a diet. You are repairing your appetite switch. You have enough to do today without adding anything else to it:

- ◆ Eat every two to three hours so that you have five feedings/day.

- ✧ Your meals can be anything as long as you have some protein.
- ✧ Snacks must not contain any sugar, flour, wheat, or simple carbs.
- ✧ Snacks must also be free of any flavor enhancer or artificial sweetener except for stevia or xylitol. That means your snack can't have any msg in it. If you plan to have soup, check the label. Some soups contain msg.

Your first weekend or day off, read Chapter 15. It will help you structure yourself so that you have less to do on your work days. Plan to shop on that day and to get things organized.

Helene came to my program as a last resort. Not only had she tried every diet known to woman, she'd given up on herself. She saw her body as her enemy. It wouldn't do what she wanted it to, and it wouldn't stop pushing her face into the Twinkies.

Even though she was a great mother and winner of the governor's award for the best teacher in the state, she felt like a failure. Her feeling of hopelessness over her eating tarnished all her successes and interfered with her enjoyment of life.

Therefore, she couldn't believe she could see evidence of

> **Test 1**
>
> - Eat every 2 or 3 hours.
> - To be counted as a legitimate meal, you must eat some protein.
> - To be counted as a legitimate snack, it must not have:
>   - Wheat
>   - Sugar
>   - Flour
>   - Artificial sweetener
>   - Msg
>   - Simple carbs

changes in her brain after only one week on Test 1. In the first place, it didn't seem like she'd done enough. She hadn't taken any food away from herself. She hadn't forced herself to eat 3 lettuce leaves waved over the vinegar bottle.

She wasn't suffering. She felt like she was eating more food than ever before, and yet. And yet. And yet, her data showed that both her NPY and her appetite were decreasing.

Did she lose weight? No. Did she care? For a change, no, because she was smart and she could see that if her appetite diminished, it couldn't help but eventually make a difference to her weight.

She said to me, "I get it. If I even lose one pound a month, in a year I'll be 12 pounds lighter."

I nodded.

"And to lose even 12 pounds a year is better than to try to lose 15 pounds in a month and to either not succeed, or to gain it back."

"Yes," I agreed. "To lose weight you won't gain back is not only much better for your health, it feels different, doesn't it?"

"I believe in myself!" The words just popped out of her mouth and her eyes got big. "I'm so surprised. I actually do believe I can do it." Tears leaked from her eyes and made her cheeks shiny.

"Of course you can. Your body has only been waiting for you to understand it. Now you can work with each other."

The To-Do List for Each Day This Week

1. Eat your three meals and two snacks.
2. Mark your chart each hour.
3. At the end of the day connect the dots
4. Answer the questions at the bottom of the chart.

5. Prepare your snacks for tomorrow and your portable breakfast, if need be.
6. Tonight put a fresh Test 1 Data Chart next to your bed.

Planning Place—Optional tool

Mealtime	Meal items	Shopping list
Breakfast		
Snack		
Lunch		
Snack		
Dinner		

FAQ and Complaints

Q Wait a minute. I feel like I'm eating too much.

A Reality check. Do you mean you're eating more regular food?

Hear me out. Are you eating more of the food that you notice when you know you are eating? Or are you eating more of the food that you ignore when you aren't conscious of what you are eating?

You know what I'm talking about right? Meals, eating during the day—this is the food that you notice you are eating. The food you eat when you're tucked into the couch watching TV, that food you *don't* notice you're eating.

Right? So is your discomfort from eating more food overall? Or is it from eating food during the part of the day when you notice what you're eating? (Only another foodie would even follow this conversation.)

If you are panicking because you are noticing that you are eating, can you put your fear into words?

Write your fear down here:

_____

_____

_____

Is this fear about the past or the future?

Would you like to take the power out of this fear? If so, use the next tool.

Relief Tool—Fear Shrinking Protocol[4]
Adapted from a technique taught and practiced by SCTRI®, Systems-Centered® Training and Research Institute.

If the fear is from the past:

1. Did something happen to you because your eating was noticed? What happened? _____

_____

2. How did you feel when that happened?_____

---
[4] The full exercises/protocols are in *the Systems-centered Training Manual*. Go to www.systemscentered.com for more information.

3. Can you pause right now and make a space inside yourself for that feeling? (Many of us try not to feel feelings like this. We try to push them away. But that doesn't actually make us feel better.)

a. Are you willing to experiment and see what will happen if you just pause and allow yourself to feel the feeling for a minute or so?

b. Keep your eyes on the experience you're having inside your body.

c. Notice if you start to tense against the feeling and relax instead.

> **I'm afraid someone will notice that I'm eating. My fear is from the past.**
> 1. My uncle used to make fun of me for eating.
> 2. It hurt my feelings. I felt bad about myself. I still do.
> 3. I'm willing to pause. The feeling is spreading all around on my insides. I feel a little sick and sort of hollow and there's a kind of vibration that feels like a slight pain in my arms and head.
> 4. I'm keeping my eyes on it. I'm noticing that it's less intense now. I can stand it more. I kind of want to punch my uncle in the mouth.
> 5. I suddenly have more energy and I feel clearer inside. I'm remembering that I'm doing this for myself and to heck with other people's stupid comments.

4. What are you noticing?
5. What are you experiencing now?

If the fear is about the future:

1. Are you thinking something that is making you afraid? What is the thought? You can write it here if you want.

_____

_____

_____

2. This thought is called a negative prediction[5]. So, reality check, do you believe you can you predict the future?

3. If you answered no, then how do you feel for yourself that you're feeling so bad from doing something you don't even believe in?

4. Is your concern less, the same, or more?

> **My fear is about the future.**
> 1. I'm afraid someone will notice that I'm eating and say something mean.
> 2. I don't think I can predict the future.
> 3. I feel sad for myself that I stopped myself this way. I'm seeing how hard I try and I really feel compassion for myself. I've got my arms around myself.
> 4. I'm feeling a lot less afraid.

If you think you can predict the future:

1. What per cent accuracy do you think you have in predicting the future? 10%, 50%, 70%, 90%

2. Whatever you circled, the opposite is your rate of being wrong about the future, which means that 90%, 50%, 30%, or 10% of the time you can't actually tell what will happen in the future.

3. Here's your choice
   a. Do you want to live in the world of the present where it's not actually scary in this moment?
   b. Do you want to live in the world of a scary future that has a certain percentage of not coming true?

> **I think I do know where trends are going.**
> 1. 50%
> 2. So 50% of the time I'm wrong.
> 3. I don't want to live in a scary future that has a 50% chance of not even happening.
> 4. I choose the present.
> 5. I'm actually feeling better just by being here now.
> 6. I'm feeling a lot less afraid.

---

[5] Borrowed from SCTRI. The full protocol is in *the Systems-centered Training Manual*, Go to www.systemscentered.com for more information.

4. Circle which world you want to live in:

    Present   Future

5. If you chose the present, how do you feel for yourself that a thought could scare you and potentially derail you from doing something really important for yourself?

6. Are you now more afraid, less afraid, or the same?

Using the Fear-Shrinking Protocol

Except when you open the door and a bear is standing right there growling at you, most fears are based on some thought. Anxieties, worries, and fears can derail us unless we know how to work with them and get to the bottom of where they're coming from.

Scary thoughts can be a instant form of time travel, taking us either to an upsetting past or a scary future. By using the protocol, we can get a bit of perspective on what we're thinking and bring ourselves back into the current reality, which is almost always less scary than the past that is over or the imaginary future.

Return to this relief tool any time you notice you've gotten off the track with the appetite switch system you're following here.

More FAQs

Q I work in a place where I'm with people all the time. How can I get my snacks? I can't leave my station.

A Wear a fanny pack or something with pockets. Make your snacks really portable and put them in your pack or pockets. (Pocket a pack of pickled peanuts.) For example, put some almonds or some grapes in your pocket. You can unobtrusively pop one into your mouth and draw no attention. (Pop a pip of pocketed peanuts.)

Q I'm afraid someone will make a comment that hurts me, like "Are you eating again?"

A Here are some responses you can use:

- o Are you being mean again? Please stop.

- o Thank you for noticing. I'm on a new diabetes prevention program and I snack every few hours. If I forget to snack tomorrow, please remind me.

- o Are you forgetting to mind your own business again?

- o Want to join me? Snacking prevents excessive appetite. Bring your own snacks. I just have enough for myself.

- o Yes, my NPY level is too high. These are special foods to fix it.

- o Yes, it's a special program to improve my brain. You might consider it yourself. (Hope it's not too late for you.)

- o This is a way I'm helping myself. If you want to support me, there's a book you can read. (*Lick It! Fix Her Appetite Switch*)

Q I keep forgetting the time.

A Set a timer on your watch or computer, or get a little portable timer and keep that in your pocket. Some have a feature that lets you set it for a certain period—like three hours—and then when it goes off, it resets to the same interval with the touch of a button.

Q Nearly four hours pass before I realize I missed my snack, and my mealtime is approaching. Do I skip the snack since I'm to lunch in another hour?

A No. Have your snack anyway. And look at the previous question. In a few weeks, your body will be trained and you'll automatically start looking for your snack at the appropriate time.

Q I sleep late on Saturday. Do I still have breakfast?

A Yes. Or you can call it lunch. I don't care what you call it, as long as you eat within one hour of awakening, and then space your meals and snacks every two to three hours.

Q I can't eat much in the morning. It makes me sick.

A One option is to have your snack as your first meal, then your breakfast as your first snack. Remember, just a handful of almonds will do.

Q I don't feel like eating when I get up.

A Congratulations, that's satiety. The only problem is that you are having it at the wrong time of day. I'll explain that in a couple of chapters. For now, notice, this is what satiety feels like. And eat something anyway.

Q If I stay up late, after having my three meals and two snacks, should I have another snack?

A You can. A good snack for evening would be milk or yogurt. If you are also a food addict, a time will come—when we deal with the addiction—that it will be important to choose an evening snack that won't trigger chain eating.

Q Sometimes I have to work a double shift. How should I space my eating?

A You will have to add some meals or snacks to keep your brain from being stressed. Continue to eat something legal every three hours.

15 The First Weekend after Training Week, Day 6

On your first day off after the end of Training Week, set aside some time for some extra planning so that you will be supporting your first eating change. If you like to be organized, you can plan your snacks for the week, get your shopping done, and get your snacks organized for the next week.

Don't plan any further than what will take you through Week 1, Day 7, because you'll be using a new test then and you'll be organizing your foods in a different way.

For the next 4 weekends (or whatever is your regular time-off schedule), set aside time to plan, shop, and organize yourself for that week's test.

Brain Trick

Here's a little brain trick. If you structure yourself to follow a practice for one month, your brain will begin to help you continue that practice. You've probably heard the saying, "21 days makes a habit."

It's actually fancier than that. Your brain is plastic. Don't worry. You aren't made of petrochemicals. It's plastic in the sense of being capable of being molded or sculptured. You can shape your brain by being intelligent about what you do and how you do it.

How Your Brain Gets Shaped

You can build new pathways in your brain. When you do a certain thing over and over, your nerves branch in a certain direction and connect with branches of other nerves that, in that part of the brain, consolidate your frequent practice so that over time the practice becomes automatic.

Practice may not make perfect, but practice does make automatic. If you create a planning, shopping, organizing routine, you'll not only get efficient at it, you'll find it easier to fit it in.

I organize my pills on Sunday morning. I line up all my vitamin and supplement bottles and drop them into little lidded boxes so that the rest of the week, they are easy to take. If I'm traveling and miss my Sunday, I have a heck of a time getting it done. On Sunday it's easy. On Monday it's nearly impossible, even if Monday is a day off.

Instead of getting mad at yourself for these tidal currents in your brain, work with them. Deliberately follow a practice, get your brain programmed, and it will become easy.

It's very hard to undo a habit. The brain doesn't like to tear down. It likes to build.

If you have brain pathways that make you thump the tree before you walk into the house, it will be hard to stop. Your neurons (nerves) are already laid out in a tree thumping pattern. You can't reach in there and rip out

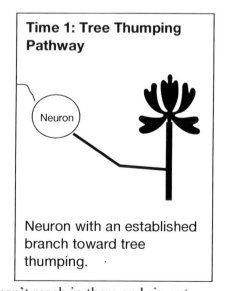

Time 1: Tree Thumping Pathway

Neuron

Neuron with an established branch toward tree thumping.

those neurons just because tree thumping is getting splinters in your knuckles.

However, if you replace tree thumping with another positive action, like leaf touching, your brain will happily build new neuron branches that promote leaf touching. Over time, leaf touching will become the preferred pathway.

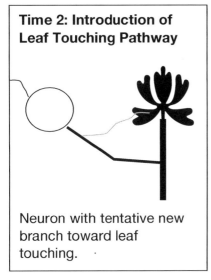

Time 2: Introduction of Leaf Touching Pathway

Neuron with tentative new branch toward leaf touching.

Let's say you have a habit of lying around Saturday morning, going out to get your car gassed up, then coming home and watching a movie.

So, build on what's already there. Put your Planning Place tool and a pencil next to the couch, and while you're lying there, reach out and fill in the blanks on the Planning Place. You will build new neuron branches that support planning.

After you fill your gas tank, continue from the station to the grocery and get your meal and snack items. After you come home from your errands, put your baggies, groceries, cutting board, and knife on the table in front of the TV, and prepare your snacks while watching your movie.

Time 3: Leaf Touching becomes the preferred pathway

Neuron with leaf touching branch stronger than tree thumping branch.

Follow this routine for a couple of months and, voila, your brain will be reprogrammed. It will then feel natural to plan your week's eating while you're lying around Saturday morning, to continue on to the grocery after you gas your car, and to divvy up your snacks while you're watching your movie.

Look at your own current Saturday (or day-off) routine and figure out how you can attach similar new actions to it.

Here is why this is so important. Snacks are consumables. You will eat them. They will get used up. If you don't have a routine for replacing them, a day will come when your pantry is empty.

The war was lost for want of a nail. The NPY target was lost for want of a snack.

It is a big deal to add two snacks a day. It is already taxing your beliefs about eating. You have a very old and entrenched belief that not eating is good. Until you see the actual results and get this pattern established, that old belief will automatically pull you away from snacking if you aren't being conscious about it.

Plus, you are already dealing with an armful of changes. You have a new daily routine, a new eating routine, and a new evening routine. This is still very fragile. An empty pantry, a missed day of snacks, and the whole thing could come tumbling down.

A regular plan for replacing snacks is key to ongoing success.

Your brain has been operating at a disadvantage for anywhere from 10 to 50 years, however long you thought you shouldn't be eating. We are one week into changing your attitude. You need more support before all this becomes automatic—as it will.

In another week you'll have some proof it works. In two more weeks you may have some dramatic proof. In three weeks, it will start being automatic and you won't care if someone is rude, mean, or ignorant. But today, today, is your chance to set yourself up for success by making absolutely sure your cupboard is never bare.

A timely snack can make all the difference between a right-sized meal and a binge. It is really, really important. The number one cause of slips and downright failure is not having snack materials close at hand.

I work underneath my kitchen. No, not in a dank hidey-hole between the

> A timely snack can make all the difference between a right-sized meal and a binge.

floorboards. My office is on the first floor. Walking up the stairs to get my snack takes 2 minutes. Do I go? No. If I don't bring my snack down when I first start writing, I am in serious danger of writing for 5 hours without leaving my chair.

It's only two minutes away, but I've missed many a snack because I tend to keep on doing whatever I'm doing.

So I work with that. I bring down my snacks and my huge water bottle. When my appetite or the alarm on my computer tells me 3 hours are up, I reach out and grab my snack. I'll mindlessly eat whatever snack is on my desk, and my NPY continues to nap.

Your snacks must be convenient. They must be ready. They must be near you when the time comes. You must have a way to replace them when they get used up.

Being diligent about this is the most important thing you can do for yourself today.

Snack Planning Tool

If you'd like to increase your success with snacking, make a list of the snacks and/or breakfast foods you will use this week. Check the items that you'll need to buy when you go out to shop today.

Breakfast	Snack	Snack	Shopping List

Weekly Planning Tool—Optional Tool

If you like making lists and you enjoy planning and structuring your time, you can use the following tool. Adapt this in the way that can work for you. If you plan to eat out for most lunches, clearly you don't need to fill in the lunch portion of the chart. You might not want to plan your dinners in advance, preferring to decide as you leave work what you feel like having. That's OK.

Feel free to ignore this tool if you feel overwhelmed by it.

Day	Mealtimes	Meal	Add to Shopping
1	Breakfast		
	Snack		
	Lunch		
	Snack		
	Dinner		
2	Breakfast		
	Snack		
	Lunch		
	Snack		
	Dinner		
3	Breakfast		
	Snack		
	Lunch		
	Snack		
	Dinner		
4	Breakfast		
	Snack		
	Lunch		
	Snack		
	Dinner		
5	Breakfast		
	Snack		
	Lunch		
	Snack		
	Dinner		
6	Breakfast		
	Snack		
	Lunch		
	Snack		
	Dinner		
7	Breakfast		
	Snack		
	Lunch		
	Snack		
	Dinner		

Organizing Your Snacks

When you get home from the grocery, pile your snack ingredients on the counter (or in front of the TV) after you've washed them. Assemble your baggies or Tupperware, cutting board, knife, and seasonings.

Divvy up the snacks into the baggies or boxes so that you have 18 separate snacks ready to go. If you want to label the bags (Monday, Tuesday, etc.), do so.

Put non-perishables, like nuts or raisins toward the end of the week. Put pre-wrapped items that won't suffer from a half day of non-refrigeration, like individually wrapped cheeses, toward the end of the week. If some snacks are already pre-packaged, like individual soup containers, they can also go toward the end of the week, so that fresh food such as strawberries, grapes, celery, salad (dressing in a separate container) can be eaten sooner and still be tasty.

Fill the 4 extra bags with foods that can be stored without refrigeration for a long time. Put one bag in your desk at home or near the place you most commonly sit. Take another bag out to your car and put it there. Put the third bag with your pile of things to take to work. Put the fourth bag in your purse.

Now you are fortified for any potential meal delay.

Organizing Breakfast

If you are not used to eating breakfast, use this day off time to organize your breakfasts for each work day. You can bake a breakfast to reheat, such as a large quiche. Or buy individual quiches (made by Nancy in the freezer section of your store, but oddly enough, not always in the breakfast section) and bake one each day. Cook up a pot of oatmeal to microwave, or divvy granola up into baggies.

Check Chapter 13 for a list of portable breakfasts.

FAQs and Complaints

Q So you're saying I don't have to plan every single meal for the rest of my life, but for sure, breakfast and snacks for the coming week.

A Yes. Being diligent about this now will pay off in a big way as this progression continues. We're programming your brain to see food planning as a normal part of your weekend. This sets you up to have the ingredients you need to be successful for Test 1, this week, and to also have a natural routine when you no longer need this book.

Q Will I always have to go to this much trouble?

A Once your brain is programmed, it won't be so much trouble. It will become part of the routine that you use to take care of yourself.

Q I don't want to have to think about food this much.

A I hear this a lot, and if you consider for a moment, this is an ironic comment. What do you think about a lot when your appetite is controlling you? Food, restaurants, and eating.

Being in recovery myself and having worked with food addicts for almost 40 years, I know how we think. We think about food and eating all the time. But we don't *notice* we're thinking about food and eating. And the way we think about food is this: we think about food as a tool that gets us comfort or relief.

This program makes you notice you're thinking about food. And it's teaching you to think about food differently—not as a tool for relief—but as a tool for relieving your driven appetite.

So the goal, now, of thinking about food, is so that you can head down an entirely different path than the path you are used to. This is why it's so uncomfortable.

We don't mind thinking about food all the time when it's part of our routine for comfort. We do mind thinking about food when it's not necessarily going to head us toward comfort.

You are going to get tools that give you comfort, but not in this way, the way that you're used to. No wonder it all feels so strange and like wearing an uncomfortable coat. This is an entirely new and different way of dealing with food.

If a part of you is reaching out her arms and saying, "Wait, wait, I want the comfort! Give me back my comfort," listen to me.

1. You are not giving up any of your comfort foods today or this week or for the next three weeks. You can use all the comfort foods as usual, just as long as they aren't your snacks. Have your comfort foods with your meals.
2. This reaction is telling you that your brain is addicted to comfort foods.
3. We'll fix this, but not now.
4. You are going to learn better ways to comfort yourself.

16 The Battle in the Brain

Adding snacks and breakfast are changes that are guaranteed to work. They *will* decrease your appetite.

> 1. Mark your chart as soon as you awaken.
> 2. Carry your chart today.
> 3. Dot each hour.
> 4. Mark all food eaten.
> 5. **Go eat breakfast.**
> 6. **Take your snacks with you.**

Looked at dispassionately, this is no big deal. We like to eat. I'm telling you to eat. I'm giving you the science that proves it's good for you. You don't even have to believe me. You have a tool (charting) that will prove to you that your appetite is shrinking.

What could be simpler? If it is simple and you have no trouble with this change, if you don't resist it, if you embrace the concept and aren't fighting it, I have great news for you. You might not be addicted to food. If so, you will have a much easier time of it and your relief from your stuck appetite switch is only 3 weeks away.

If, however, you are wrestling with this process, if you want to argue with each point, are forgetting your snacks or missing your snack times over and over, and not using the tips that will make your food available or remind you to eat, you are probably addicted to food.

That's the bad news.

The good news is that there's a way out and you'll be shocked at how different you will feel and how clear your mind will become after we've dealt with the addiction.

Considering our last umpteen decades have been organized around eating—thinking about food, wanting food, planning to hit certain drive-through, concealing eating, protecting our stash—it's amazing how awkward it is to add two mere snacks a day.

Partly it's odd because we aren't used to noticing we're eating. It's this big secret we've been keeping from ourselves. Clandestine eating, pretending to ourselves we're not eating, or telling ourselves we deserve certain foods because of the day we've had—these are all ways we've slid past full consciousness of what we're actually doing.

But something else is also going on. We are hearing from one of the major causes of a stuck appetite switch—the addicted brain. Even though we're not actually doing anything this week to challenge the food addiction—we're not taking away any foods, we're not restricting any comfort foods—the part of the brain that is addicted is having a fit.

The more you have to wrestle with yourself to make this one simple change, the more likely it is that you are addicted to food and your brain isn't happy with this new system. It doesn't *want* your appetite to decrease. It doesn't want *anything* to get in the way of the comfort system that is guaranteed to work. Just doing the charting and becoming more conscious is getting in the way of the habit of avoidance that the addictive brain has nurtured.

It's as though we have two selves, two people inside us. One of our inner selves wants desperately to be happy, to feel comfortable in her skin, to have more energy, to move more easily, to feel good about her body, to be healthier. The other inner self wants to avoid reality, crawl into her cocoon, and stay safe. Comfort foods do this for her, and she'll fight anyone or anything that threatens her use of these foods.

It's not a fair fight. Your brain is layered. The parts on the top are more conscious. The deeper, lower parts are less conscious. The deeper in the brain a function is, the more power it has to overrule the higher layers.

The decisions made by the part of you that wants to feel better, have better health, and possibly look better, are higher in your brain than the addicted part of you. Notice that the addicted part of the brain is way down there, within the reactive, non-thinking part of the brain, and close to survival functioning. When someone messes with your addiction, it can feel like a threat to your survival, and you will fight it with all the energy you'd use to pull yourself out of dangerous waters.

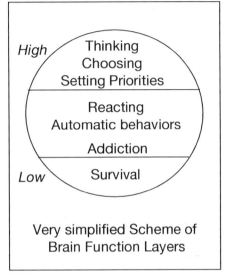

Very simplified Scheme of Brain Function Layers

Have you ever had someone try to monitor your food or eating? How did you react? Did you say, "Thank you so much. I've been having trouble with this."

I doubt it. If you didn't blow them out of the water, I'm guessing you fortified your secret stash within hours.

When you are on your way to your very favorite restaurant and the traffic department has blocked a lane so that it takes an hour to travel ten feet, do you say, "Oh well, that restaurant isn't that important, I'll just go a different way and get a salad instead," or do you either continue toward that restaurant or think of another one that has almost the same foods?

If your boss says something that feels threatening to your security, do you take a nice long walk, talk to three friends, and meditate for about an hour or do you skip the salad and go straight for the fat-starch combo?

When comfort food feels *essential* to your survival, anything that gets in the way of obtaining it is perceived as a *threat* to survival. We can even, hold on to your hat, *create* threats in order to have a reason to eat. Any time we give ourselves too much to do, hold to impossible standards of accomplishment, work too long, become too perfectionistic, we put ourselves into a threatened state to which the solution is eating.

So, these two little innocent snacks are like red flags to a bull. Your addiction will read their potential accurately, as a threat to its happy sedated state. It may even have a fit over the charting, not wanting you to become more aware of what you are doing.

We like to think we are sentient creatures in full mastery of our choices, but any addict will tell you that the addiction is sneaky, powerful, cunning, tricky, conniving, and relentless.

What can we do about this?

Here are some of your options.

1. We have an incredible bargain in that the very most successful program for addiction is free. More addicts have found liberation and rewarding lives from anonymous 12-step programs than any other treatment program. In fact, many paid programs depend on 12-step programs as their primary, long-term aftercare program. For us, the top choices are Overeaters Anonymous, Food Addicts Anonymous, Eating Addicts Anonymous, and Compulsive Eaters Anonymous. Each has a website and each has strengths and weaknesses which I detail in my book, *How to Make Almost Any Diet Work*. In that book you'll also find tools that combine the

best of each of these organizations by updating some of the routine parts of meetings to take into account recent research.

2. Replace comfort chemicals triggered by food with relief chemicals from sources other than food. More about this later.

3. Practice Powerlessness. It may seem counter-intuitive that admitting powerlessness should be a weapon against addiction, but millions have proved its effectiveness.

The brain chemistry involved explains this. When we try hard, we activate a brain chemical called norepinephrine (NE). Most overeaters have an extra abundance of NE going to the binge center of the brain (hypothalamus). They got this additional wiring from two sources, from early childhood stress and/or from trying too hard.

Here's the catch-22 that's embedded in dieting. Dieting requires that we try hard. We try not to eat certain things. We try to eat a lot less of something. We try to change everything about our eating in a matter of days. We try to tolerate being hungry. We try to make ourselves like less interesting food. We try to make ourselves exercise. We try not to bite off the head of a person stupid enough to eat a brownie in front of us while we're on a diet.

All this trying causes a flood of NE to our binge center. And NE activates. It stimulates. When it floods the binge center, it stimulates appetite. It's a no-win scenario. Trying hard will inevitably trigger binging.

Any time you are trying hard, you are activating your binge center. You *will* eventually eat.

Admitting powerlessness is the antidote to trying hard. When we recognize the truth—that we are powerlessness over addiction, including the deep-seated chemical process in the brain that is the addicted part of our selves—it gives us immeasurable relief. Of course it's stronger than we are. Of course it always wins.

Are you curious about what will happen if you practice powerlessness?

1. Sit in a chair that allows you to keep both feet on the ground and supports you in an aligned position.
2. Bring yourself to a more centered place by tuning into your breathing.
3. Notice the experience of breathing in.
4. Notice the experience of breathing out.
5. Pause just a bit at the end of your exhale and notice that you are offered a little window into yourself.
6. After several breaths, say, "I am powerless over eating."
7. Remain quiet for a few minutes.
8. Notice what happens.
9. Pause again and let your awareness have some room.
10. Take a break before reading the next chapter, which leaps back into the left side of the brain.

17 Meanwhile, Back at the Testing Center

After seven days of Test 1, you will begin Test 2. Test 2 will tell you if you need to activate polypeptide YY.

PYY is a satiety chemical. It makes you lose interest in eating.

Hard to imagine, I know, but one day you'll get bored with lifting that fork and want to do something else. It will happen so seamlessly, you might not notice that an earth-shaking event has just transformed your life. But at some point, you'll look back and realize that you lost interest in food and left the eating place because you were attracted to another activity. That, my dear, is satiety.

You're going to love PYY. It's an incredibly helpful brain chemical. It lowers your appetite, it increases your metabolism, and it gets you interested in moving your body.

What a deal!

If you are deficient in PYY or your body is not processing it, then you must do what builds it up. Once you have enough PYY, then all you have to do to keep your supply going is to never skip a meal. You've already heard me harp on this. Don't skip a meal. Don't ever skip breakfast. Blah, blah, blah.

Hey, if it weren't important, I wouldn't emphasize it. It's really, really important. By not ever skipping or delaying a meal, you prevent NPY, you preserve PYY, and you also shelve a bunch of other chemicals that are triggered by meal-skipping, including chemicals that make you store fat and are resistant to ever burning that fat again.[6]

I'm telling you, your body is defended against starvation. You have an entire army that will fight to make you eat if you skip meals. You absolutely cannot resist this army. It will win.

And haven't you proved this to yourself over and over? Haven't you been driven to eat when in your deepest heart, you didn't want to be?

Test 2 will reveal recovery of PYY functioning and an increase in satiety. Increased satiety will cause decreased appetite.

One part of your brain is not happy with this information. Guess who? The addicted brain does not want you to reach satiety. It wants you to skip meals so that you'll be set up to eat.

It will complain that fixing snacks and remembering to eat them is too much trouble. Never mind that you'd drive 10 miles out of your way or lose an hour of your day to get a particular comfort food. That 3 minutes spent putting grapes in a baggy will seem like an ordeal.

Whenever your brain starts telling you this stuff, that's your addicted brain and it is out to sabotage you. Distract it. Sit down and do the practice of powerlessness from the previous chapter or go online and read something on the www.oa.org website. Buy a copy of *The 12 Steps and 12 Traditions of Overeaters Anonymous* and read a couple paragraphs

---

[6] If you would like the details—the names of the chemicals, the process, the science—get my book called *How to Make Almost Any Diet Work*. That's a resource if more information will strengthen you. (It's written in the same style as this book, with sass and charts to make it easier to understand.)
You won't have to read the entire book. In this Appendix, you'll find a guide that will help you go straight to the info you're interested in in *How to Make Almost Any Diet Work*.

when your brain starts feeding you such bunk.

Get savvy. Notice thoughts from your addicted brain and begin the habit of interrupting it. As you work with yourself, building a new brain pathway that reaches for recovery, you'll weaken the neuron pathway that leads to your food addiction. It will get easier to let go and feel the comfort of powerlessness. It will begin to feel heart-filling to read the stories of other recovering people. You'll start to release other comforting brain chemicals that aren't associated with eating.

And guess what will happen? It will get easy to drop some grapes into a baggie.

Work with yourself to weaken the addicted path and strengthen the recovery path.

18 Preparing for Test 2

Satiety shuts off your appetite switch. PYY is an important player in that process. Test 2 will reveal if you have been deficient in PYY (and were missing other steps in the satiety process).

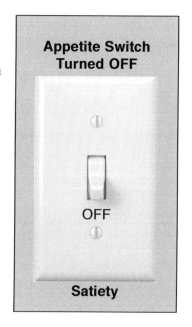

If you've never been a meal skipper, then most likely your PYY is fine, but if you're a skipper, your PYY functioning could be taking a deep nap.

Meal skipping causes PYY production to shut down. Without PYY, it is hard to reach satiety.

It only makes sense. If you are victimized by periodic famine, then of course your body wants you to be obsessed with eating. It will suppress PYY.

You've got to love this about the brain. It wants to be healthy. Given half a chance, the brain starts to repair itself right away if it has the ingredients to make the repair. With Test 2, we'll find out if the brain seizes the opportunity to repair itself. You'll give your brain the elements it needs to restore PYY.

Brain repair requires steady supplies of blood sugar and protein. This means that your blood sugar must become more even and your blood must be chock full of amino acids, the components of protein.

In Test 2 you will provide both conditions by upgrading your snacks. Snacks will now consist of 50% protein and 50% complex carbohydrates

If this makes a difference in the data you collect, you'll know that a lack of PYY was part of your appetite switch problem and that by converting Test 2 to Change 2, you'll always have PYY (and other satiety chain reactions) protecting you from overeating.

Preparation for Test 2

1. To prepare for Test 2, lay in supplies of portable proteins and complex carbs. Rule 3 still applies.
2. By the end of Week 1, Day 7, have enough 50-50 snack foods to last until your next day off or weekend.

Rules
Rule 1. Make each change in order
Rule 2. Make one change and only one change this week.
Rule 3. Snacks must not have:
    a. Wheat
    b. Sugar
    c. Flour
    d. Artificial sweetener
    e. Msg
    f. Simple carbs
Stevia and xylitol are OK.

3. Make 7 copies of the Test 2 Data Chart.
4. The night before the first day of Test 2, put a Test 2 Data Chart next to your bed so it will be there for you to mark in the morning.
5. On your next day off or weekend, follow your new structure for making your work week easier.
6. Keep an eye on resistance from your addicted brain. If it bothers you,

use one of your tools to handle it.

50-50 snacks

Any food that is listed by itself is a natural 50-50 snack. For example, milk has a enough milk sugar and soy nuts have enough protein to be good enough. Same goes with all nuts, except your nutty aunt who is all protein.

Milk	Soy milk (unsweetened)
Soy nuts	Banana and yogurt
Cheese and apple	Almonds
Peanuts	Pickle and sliced beef roll-ups
V8 juice and cheese curds	Artichoke hearts and peanuts
Pineapple and cottage cheese	Asparagus and ham
Feta and olives	String cheese and spaghetti sauce
Beef barley soup	Chicken and wild rice soup
Celery and peanut butter (all natural, no sweetener)	Apple stuffed with cottage cheese or peanut butter and a couple of raisins
Cheddar cheese and corn on the cob	Oatmeal and peanut butter
Tomato stuffed with tuna	Tuna mixed with celery and grapes
Shrimp cocktail	Caesar salad (no croutons)
Corned beef and cabbage	

Test 2 Chart

Basic Data--Test 2										Circle Wake-up Time								Date				
	Time of Day	5	6	7	8	9	10	11	12	**1**	**2**	**3**	**4**	**5**	**6**	**7**	**8**	**9**	10	11	12	1	2	3	4
Appetite	Can't stop																								
	More food																								
	Craving food																								
	Food focused																								
	Quiet																								
Hunger	Starved																								
	Strong																								
	Moderate																								
	Mild																								
	Not hungry																								
Eating	Protein																								
	Comp carb																								
	Simp carb																								
	Fat/oil																								
Caffeine	Yes																								
Satiety	Not satisfied																								
	Satisfied																								
Sress	High																								
	Medium																								
	Low																								
	None																								

Mark the following items just once each day. You can use a mark or make a note for your answer.

Sleep Problems		Felt like exercising.	Yes	No	

19 Week 2, Test 2

The To-Do List Each Day This Week

1. Eat your three meals and two 50-50 snacks.
2. Mark your chart each hour.
3. At the end of the day connect the dots
4. Answer the questions at the bottom of the chart.
5. Prepare your snacks for tomorrow and your portable breakfast, if need be.
6. Each night put a fresh Test 2 Data Chart next to your bed.
7. On your first weekend or day off, structure your food so that the coming work week will be easier.

As I was driving home today, I noticed that cows with their little offspring were ambling along a narrow path from one pasture to another. No human was involved. Somehow they had been programmed to change fields at a certain time of day. I'm guessing that those little heifers will have the routine down by the time they are leading cow babies of their own.

I thought, if a cow's brain can learn a pattern, surely we brilliant humans can too. And you are well on your way. By following this practice of pausing each hour to notice your body, and by eating every two to three hours, your brain has already begun constructing pathways to make this a routine. In another week, it will be much easier. Soon it will be automatic.

> **Test 2**
> 1. Eat every 2 or 3 hours.
> 2. To be counted as a legal meal, you must eat some protein.
> 3. To be counted as a legal snack, it must be 50% protein and 50% complex carb. It must *not* have:
>   - a. Wheat
>   - b. Sugar
>   - c. Flour
>   - d. Artificial sweetener
>   - e. Msg
>   - f. Simple carbs

If a cow can do it, so can I.

20 Analyzing Data from Test 1

All the Data Analysis chapters are in the Appendices. The Test 1 analysis process is in Appendix B. You can begin analyzing the Test 1 data now or you can wait till all the tests have been completed and immerse yourself in the analysis of all 5 tests together.

You have options.
1. If you've already noticed that your appetite has decreased, and you don't want to get involved with data analysis, continue to the next chapter.
2. If you want to see what the figures show, go to Appendix B and start the process.
3. If you get overwhelmed as you start working in Appendix B, and you already feel trusting of this process and are planning to continue with it, move on to the next chapter.
4. If you can tolerate some minimal data analysis and have some interest in seeing what the figures show, continue through Appendix B, Part 1, then return to the next chapter.
5. If you love data analysis and you want to learn everything you

can about your appetite switch, proceed through Appendix B as far as you want to go.

21 Meanwhile, Back at Test 2

Whether you stepped out to analyze Test 1 or you arrived here from the previous chapter, you are in the midst of Test 2. This is your third week learning this new system and your second week of change.

Test 2 is but a refinement on Test 1, defining legal snacks as being 50% protein and 50% complex carbohydrate. For seven days you will give yourself this test and keep records using Test 2 charts.

How are you feeling about charting? Some people find it supports them in checking in with themselves and eating their snacks and meals in a timely fashion.

Others hate it and it gets in their way. Do you think you'd keep the changes and tests going if you weren't charting? If you hate dotting but see some value in it, a simpler chart measuring the most important indicators is on the next page. Switch to the Bare Bones Chart for Test 3.

Some continue dotting, even if they don't intend to analyze the data, because it reminds them to check in with their bodies. If you do like learning about your body, chart until you complete Test 3. That test will show you how much more of a difference that chemical makes to your appetite switch. You'll also discover how this chemical affects hunger.

It's your choice. What matters most of all is keeping this system manageable so that you'll continue to learn it. If charting promotes your learning and your confidence in yourself, then it has value. If charting is such a drag that you want to throw the whole process out, then stopping it is wise.

Bare Bones Chart												Circle Wake-up Time							Date				
	Time of Day	5	6	7	8	9	10	11	12	**1**	**2**	**3**	**4**	**5**	**6**	**7**	**8**	**9**	10	11	12	1	2	3	4
Appetite	Can't stop																								
	More food																								
	Craving food																								
	Food focused																								
	Quiet																								
Eating	Protein																								
	Comp carb																								
	Simp carb																								
	Fat/oil																								
Tryptophan-1 dot/unit																									
Sress	High																								
	Medium																								
	Low																								
	None																								

22 The Magic Pill

What if there were a food you could eat that would help you relax, reduce your pain, protect you from mean people, decrease your appetite, make you less vulnerable to addiction, reduce your hunger, help you to eat more slowly, and tell you when you've had enough food?

Wouldn't you just want to go right out and get it? Well there is such a food—in fact more than one—and eating sufficient amounts of it will be your next test. If you are still charting, you may be curious to see the degree of change you will document when you eat this food.

Are you a quart low already?

Field Serotonin Test

Check the statements that are mostly true or true more often than not.

	Statements	Yes
1	When someone is rude to you, it doesn't bother you.	
2	You can feel bad even when a stranger is mean to another stranger.	
3	You tend to eat slowly	
4	When someone is rude to you, it gnaws at you for hours.	

5	You stop eating as soon as you feel full.	
6	A tease that's just a little hurtful worries you, even if you know it isn't true.	
7	After you start eating, you usually feel full in 30 to 45 minutes.	
8	You tend to eat quickly.	
9	If someone teases you, even if they were a little mean, you tease them right back,.	
10	You can eat for hours before feeling full.	
11	You recover quickly after something is stressful.	
12	You feel stressed most of the time, even when nothing is really wrong.	
13	You fall asleep fairly easily.	
14	Most of the time you aren't aware of your dreams.	
15	You felt safe as a child.	
16	People have called you clumsy.	
17	People consider you to be mellow.	
18	You're afraid of mean, sarcastic, or hostile people.	
19	You are easily pleased.	
20	Things have to be just right before you are pleased, and even then you don't exactly experience pleasure.	
21	You've been called thin-skinned or too sensitive.	
22	You can be hurt when someone is thoughtless, even when you're pretty sure they didn't intend to hurt you.	
23	You get depressed.	
24	If you take anti-depressants, sometimes they don't seem to work as well as at other times.	
25	Sometimes your hunger just won't quit.	
26	You still remember that Uncle Unfair slighted you 15 years ago.	
27	Some things happened when you were a child that you didn't know how to handle.	

Look back over your answers. Are your checks mostly associated with the shaded rows? If so, then you have natural insulation against stress and mean or thoughtless people.

Are your checks mostly associated unshaded rows? Then you are have insufficient supplies of a neurochemical that can protect you from hurtful people and stress.

That neurochemical is serotonin. When you have enough of it, it does a lot of good in so many ways it's miraculous.

The Pursuit of Comfort

It's safe to say that we pursue comfort. We do this in part because we are more stressed than the average person. We may or may not actually have more to handle than other folks, but either they aren't stressed by as many things that stress us, or it lingers longer with us than it does with them.

When I was a graduate student, my advisor rejected my first outline of my master's thesis with a comment akin to, "You'll never amount to anything." My very next memory after reading his criticism was eating Minnie Pearl fried chicken. I have no memory of getting from the college to the restaurant or of anything else that happened that day.

My husband of the time said blithely, "Just rewrite it."

Rewrite it? Like it's simple? My entire future is at the bottom of a strip mine and he's waving his arm like he's batting away a moth. Of course it wasn't happening to him, but I'd seen him sail through similar challenges as if it were a normal part of living.

He amazed me by being relaxed most of the time. He didn't drive himself the way I did, yet he accomplished the same course work and got good grades. He was easily pleased.

You and I, on the other hand, most likely started our lives with one of two situations:
- With a built-in vulnerability that caused us to feel slights more keenly, meanness more deeply, and to be more susceptible to emotional pain.
- Inside a family that caused pain.

If we really lost the birth lottery, we started out with both conditions.

We had to figure out how to cope and our first efforts were to get ourselves more serotonin. We sure were smart. Of course we didn't know we were after serotonin, but when we ate sugar or starches to feel better, that's what we got.

Over time, other brain chemicals got involved, but at first, what soothed us was serotonin.

Unfortunately, if we were either thin-skinned or in a mean family—or both—we turned to the well so often it went dry. And the next thing that happened is that we started eating too much.

We ate too much because we'd used up nature's most effective satiety chemical. Serotonin had been soothing us, yes, but it had also made us stop eating when we'd had enough. Once we'd used it up, we lost our regulator.

Many other chemical changes proceeded from there, creating other annoying conditions such as:

- Clumsiness
- Depression
- Vulnerability to addiction
- Vulnerability to PTSD
- Non-stop hunger
- Difficulty relaxing
- Tendencies to try too hard
- Vulnerability to pain
- Susceptibility to hopelessness or giving up

I get stressed just thinking about it.

Fortunately there's something we can do about this. We can replace the serotonin. When we do, it can reverse many of those conditions, although it won't necessarily give us a nicer birth family. It will, however, give us more of a Teflon coating so that nasty comments slide off.

Replacing your serotonin is Test 3. If you notice a difference in vulnerability after a couple of weeks, you've hit the jackpot. You now have a very effective remedy for stress, *as long as you keep this change going.*

It's very important to remember that this chemical gets used up and it has to be replaced or you'll return to your former over-exposed self.

You can also evaluate your Test 3 charts and find out what they show. Some indicators may be subtle initially, so the charts may show more progress than you can actually detect with the naked eye.

Serotonin Pre-Test

Question						
Are you generally hungry when you wake up?	Yes			No		
At what time of day are you most vulnerable to chain eating?[7]						
How long does a chain eating episode typically last? (In hours)	.5	1	1.5	2	2.5	3+
What foods do you eat when you chain eat? Circle any combination that is typical for you.	Fruit Veg Protein Complex carb			Sweet Starch Fat Salt		
Have you noticed a relationship between feeling stressed and chain eating?	Yes			No		
When you are stressed, does your chain eating typically increase or decrease?	Decrease			Increase		
How would you rate your average level of stress in the last week?	Low		Med		High	
How vulnerable did you feel the last few days? Was your degree of vulnerability:	Low		Med		High	
How relaxed have you been lately?	Very		Some		Not	
How have you been sleeping?	Soundly		Slightly disturbed		Very disturbed	

---

[7] Chain eating is eating one thing after another; for example, eating dinner, then a sweet, then a sweet-fat combination, then a starch, then something else.

Preparing for Test 3

1. Check the list of foods that increase your body's serotonin (ST).
2. Lay in a supply of those foods before Week 3 begins.
3. Make 7 copies of the Test 3 chart.
4. Plan to continue 50-50 snacks until Test 3 is completed.

Tryptophan Sources that Increase ST

Turkey

Milk

Sesame seeds

Tahini

Sesame oil

Soy milk

Parmesan

Mozzarella

Pumpkin seeds

Test 3 Chart

Notice that there's a new row, inserted beneath the Eating category. This category is called tryptophan, because this is the amino acid that your brain will use for manufacturing serotonin. Every time you eat 1 unit of tryptophan, put a dot in that row at the time that you eat it.

As important as it is to eat tryptophan-rich foods, it matters also to make sure you are getting enough. Effective results are dependent on getting a sufficient dose.

Basic Data--Test 3											Circle Wake-up Time									Date					
	Time of Day	5	6	7	8	9	10	11	12	1	2	3	4	5	6	7	8	9	10	11	12	1	2	3	4
Appetite	Can't stop																								
	More food																								
	Craving food																								
	Food focused																								
	Quiet																								
Hunger	Starved																								
	Strong																								
	Moderate																								
	Mild																								
	Not hungry																								
Eating	Protein																								
	Comp carb																								
	Simp carb																								
	Fat/oil																								
Tryptophan-1 dot/unit																									
Caffeine	Yes																								
Satiety	Not satisfied																								
	Satisfied																								
Sress	High																								
	Medium																								
	Low																								
	None																								
Mark the following items just once each day. You can use a mark or make a note for your answer.																									
Sleep Problems				**Felt like exercising.**						**Yes**			**No**												

Test 3

Eat or drink at least 4 units of tryptophan per day for at least five days of Week 3. (***Do not apply these units to any medications, pills, or homeopathic remedies that you take***. The units in this book are a measure I devised to make your job easier and they apply to the following foods only.)

Units of Tryptophan

Food	1 Unit	4 Units
Turkey-white meal	1 ounce	4 ounces
Turkey-dark meat	1.5 ounces	6 ounces
Turkey-packaged breast lunch meat	2 ounces	8 ounces
Milk-whole	4.5 ounces	18 ounces
Milk-low fat	7 ounces	29 ounces
Yogurt	11 ounces	44 ounces
Sesame seeds	1 ounce	4 ounces
Tahini	1 ounce	4 ounces
Sesame oil	1 ounce	4 ounces
Soy milk	5.5 ounces	23 ounces
Mozzarella	Bit more than half ounce	2 1/3 oz.
Parmesan	2/3 oz.	2.5 oz.
Ricotta	2.5 ounces	10 ounces
Cottage cheese	2.5 oz.	10 oz.
Pumpkin seeds	1 oz	4 oz.

FAQ

Q Do I have to eat all 4 units at one time during the day?

A No. You can have a glass of milk at breakfast and then 3 ounces of turkey for lunch.

Q I like chicken better than turkey. Can I just have chicken?

A Chicken, for some reason, doesn't deliver tryptophan to the brain in the same way that turkey does. All meats and most protein foods contain some measure of tryptophan, but turkey is the all round best source for the brain's use.

I can prove this to you. After Thanksgiving dinner, do you want to take a nap? How about after a chicken dinner, do you get as sleepy as you do at Thanksgiving? The traditional American Thanksgiving meal is an almost perfect tryptophan delivery system and one of the first effects of tryptophan delivery to the brain is feeling more relaxed or sleepy.

Q I've looked up tryptophan values in some other foods and they seem comparable to milk and turkey. Can I substitute other foods?

A You can if you don't like the ones listed here, but all of the foods in the above list seem to provide superior tryptophan delivery to the brain and of these, milk and turkey are the best. I can't find an explanation for this and I've been searching for years. I'm guessing there's some enzyme or micro-nutrient that we either haven't measured or haven't yet discovered that is influencing tryptophan delivery in turkey and milk.

Q Can't I just take a serotonin pill?

A Even if there were a serotonin pill, it wouldn't cross into the brain, so it wouldn't do you any good.

Q What about taking a tryptophan pill?

A Although 5-HTP can be useful when traveling, I don't advise it as a long term solution. Long term use of 5-HTP (5-Hydroxytryptophan) may reduce your D2 receptors and you don't want that happening. Lack of D2 receptors may have made you vulnerable to food addiction in the first place. Also, it's contraindicated for people taking anti-depressants and not recommended for pregnant women.

Q OK, I'll just use the pills when I'm traveling. How much should I take?

A Look on the bottle. **The units in the above Units of Tryptophan table do not apply to pills or medications.** Those food units are a measure I devised myself to simplify your job when you're shopping or cooking.

Q 4 ounces seems like a lot of turkey. Can I just eat 1 ounce a day? I don't like the other choices.

A The effectiveness of Test 3 depends on getting enough tryptophan into your system to make an appreciable difference in your brain serotonin. 1 ounce of turkey won't do it. Success here is quite dose dependent.

Q I'm a vegetarian and lactose intolerant. What shall I do?

A Use tahini, soy milk, sesame, and pumpkin seeds to get your tryptophan. Pumpkin and sesame seeds count as a 50-50 snack. My body reacts positively right away to a glass of unsweetened soy milk.

Q There must be something to the warm milk at night remedy.

A Yes. Warming milk does provide better tryptophan delivery.

Q I started this and I had a lot of vivid dreams.

A When people start replenishing their serotonin, vivid dreaming does often occur.

Q Can I get too much food tryptophan?

A Serotonin gets used up fast, every time you are stressed. Unless you have a completely relaxing life and are rarely challenged, you're going through serotonin like grease through a goose.

   My main concern is that you not burn out on tryptophan-rich foods. Since the choices for good delivery foods are limited, I wouldn't want you to have so much turkey that you would never want to eat it again.

   After Week 3 is over, you'll find out how to handle Change 3 if you need to incorporate it. For now, stick to 20 units for Week 3.

23 Week 3, Test 3

The test you'll be taking this week is one of the most important. Serotonin insufficiency is a major cause of overeating. Serotonin, unlike PYY, affects both appetite *and* hunger.

When you don't have enough serotonin, not only will your appetite be more bothersome, you'll also be hungrier. Serotonin (or the lack of it) affects you much more than you may realize. It regulates how fast you eat. It influences your food choices. It determines how quickly you feel full.

It calms you down. It makes you feel less vulnerable, and it makes you somewhat less prone to compulsive behavior. If you have good serotonin functioning when you are a child, it gives you some protection from incompetent parents, and should you be faced with a trauma, it will help you get over it.

Not having well-functioning serotonin in childhood sets you up to become addicted to something. If food is your primary addiction, congratulations. You found a route that still allowed you to have a decent life. Food addiction costs, to be sure, but your other choices—alcohol, drugs, gambling, sex—are hell on a lifestyle.

Once you are addicted, serotonin can still help, by reducing the stress that triggers eating. So this week is important for you. It may explain why you've had to struggle all your life.

You know the drill. Have that T3 chart next to your bed when you wake up in the morning. Keep it with you all day and check yourself every hour. Remember to dot the tryptophan row every time you have a unit of tryptophan.

Dot your Test 3 charts for seven days, and then you can rest for a bit.

> **Test 3**
> 1. Eat every 2 or 3 hours.
> 2. To be counted as a legitimate meal, you must eat some protein.
> 3. To be counted as a legal snack, it must be 50% protein and 50% complex carb. It must *not* have:
>   a. Wheat
>   b. Sugar
>   c. Flour
>   d. Artificial sweetener (except stevia)
>   e. Msg
>   f. Simple carbs
> 4. Eat 20 units of tryptophan throughout week 3. (That's 4 units a day for five days.)

First Hill-Almost Done

As you approach the end of Week 3, you will be 60% through the process of turning off your appetite switch. If this were a footrace, you'd be on the down-slope of the first hill, with just one more hill to climb.

FAQ

Q Why do I have to keep the snacks going? I tested them and they didn't make a difference.

A Three reasons.

- You may not have given your PYY long enough to recover. Keeping Test 2 going while you are undertaking Test 3 gives your PYY a better chance.

- o Serotonin may help your PYY recover.
- o It's easier to see what difference serotonin makes when those other appetite switch influences are already being managed.

Q Do I have to eat my units 5 days in a row?
A No. Any 5 days within the week are good.

Q Can I eat 5 units for four days?
A Yes.

Q Can I eat 3 units every day?
A Yes.

Q Can I just take pills?
A See the previous chapter.

Q I stopped using the charts, but now I'm interested. If I don't have Week 2 charts, will it do me any good to keep charts for Week 3?
A Yes. Go ahead and use the T3 charts.

Q I'm sick of charting. How long will this go on?
A Next week, you can stop charting. When we do test 5, you might want to chart afterwards to see the results. Of course if charting is souring you on the whole process, I'd rather you forget charting and learn the system anyway.

Charting is a tool. If it helps keep you conscious, it's useful. If it is just too much, it isn't.

24 Homesick?

We have lots of chemicals bouncing around in our brains, balancing each other or fighting each other. For almost a month, you have been paying attention to the major players that make the appetite switch work correctly.

If you've been following this process faithfully, you've decreased a voracious chemical, increased a satisfied-with-the-meal chemical, and are this week working on the closest thing overeaters have to a Magic Pill. (Although, as warned in a previous chapter, taking it in food form is much better for you in the long run than actually taking a pill.)

About now, you may be getting tired of the whole process and just want to go back to eating the way you used to. If I say one little thing to bother you, you are vulnerable to saying, "That's it! This isn't working for me."

Why would that happen, especially now when you are almost through? Why would you want to quit when you're mere days away from construction of new brain connections that will make all this easier for you? What is putting such thoughts in your head?

Here are some of the possibilities:

Homesick

This was exciting at first—the guarantee of something that could make a difference, the newness, having hope for a first time in a long time. But then, it turned out you had to do something, something that was different from what you are used to.

Never underestimate the power of the familiar. It's what makes women stay with abusive men. It makes us hesitant to leave a terrible job for riskier work that would be much more fulfilling. It makes us hang on to a house that's too expensive or a geography that we've outgrown.

One of the greatest documents ever written is the *Declaration of Independence.* I find it expresses well the dilemma of leaving the warm but confining womb of addiction.

> **From the Declaration of Independence**
> ...accordingly, all experience hath shewn that mankind are more disposed to suffer, while evils are sufferable, than to right themselves by abolishing the forms to which they are accustomed.

The familiar is, in itself, soothing. After prolonged strangeness, it calls even more loudly.

Once upon a time, I was walking down a street in Istanbul. I was weary from strangeness, from being surrounded by a harsh male-dominated world, from holes in the floor instead of toilets, from water unsafe to drink, from religious buildings that forbid women, and I came across a McDonalds. I felt enormous relief.

I went in, got a hamburger, and just sat there. And for a change, despite being a food addict, it wasn't about the food. In fact, I have no memory of the taste of it, and I remember tastes, including the first Heath bar I ate when I was five. No, this comfort was from the familiar, from the golden arches of home.

The familiar draws us with considerable power.

You may be experiencing a similar thing here. At first this was an exotic foreign country but now you just want to be home—and the feeling of home can be delivered by the old eating.

A chemical causes this. It will pass. Read on.

I'm bored with the whole thing.

Ennui or boredom is usually a consequence of being removed from the addictive substance, and it's one of the experiences we have when certain nerves aren't being fired due to a decrease in a neurotransmitter.

Translation: the changes you have already made are causing decreased stimulation of the addicted part of your brain. Those neurons want some excitement. They don't hurt yet (craving) but they are uncomfortable.

This is too much trouble.

I don't want to have to think about food all the time. I just want to live my life.

I've had that feeling myself, and what I've learned is this—that longing for freedom is akin to the feeling I've had when I've had other conditions that separate me from what most people are able to do.

When I had to wear a leg brace after a hamstring injury, I envied people who could just get into a car and drive, without taking 10 minutes to wedge themselves into the seat. When I had a debilitating bout with chemical sensitivity, I envied people who could go to movies or restaurants or stay in hotels as if it were a simple and easy thing to do.

The reality is, if you are a food addict, you have a disability. This disability separates you from the normal non-addicted person. (Although in America, being addicted is probably the norm. We have a lifestyle that foments addiction.)

Like any disability, food addiction makes some things easier and many things harder. As you pull yourself into more recovery, that begins to reverse. Eventually many things will be easier and some things harder.

You are in the second hardest phase of recovery, the part where everything is hard and not much is easy. If you will hang on and keep taking each step one-at-a-time, things should lighten up in a few days. And if you keep going, you will be coming out of all the hardest phases in about two weeks.

I'm disappointed to realize I have to keep these changes going.

I agree. It's hard when this realization sinks in. We want recovery to work like aspirin, to take two and be better in the morning.

Coming out of denial is painful. I remember when I realized my beloved grandmother was never going to get younger. Every time I visited her, she'd lost a little bit of some capacity. It hit me one day—how she was that day was the best she would ever be, that the next time I visited, something else would be lost.

Before I could enjoy what she still had, I had to mourn the reality that she was losing ground. I did mourn that reality, and then I could appreciate what I still had of her and could immerse myself in our relationship.

Make room in yourself for your sadness, anger, grief, or disappointment due to the reality that you have a condition that requires ongoing attention. Pause, still yourself, and make plenty of internal room.

If you notice that you are tense inside, trying to push against the experience in your body, relax. Relax around the feeling.

If you notice your fists tightening like you want to punch somebody, or your feet wanting to kick, go ahead, punch the air, kick out—just don't hurt yourself or anything or anyone else. Allow that angry energy to release itself. Notice that it's energy and that energy feels good. Energy is life-giving. Allow it.

The Internal Saboteur

How many diet books have you actually read to the last page? How many food plans have you been able to sustain? What interrupted you, do you know? Most likely it was the addicted part of the brain, getting uncomfortable.

Those first stirrings of protest from the addicted brain are showing up in all of the above symptoms. Yes, what you are feeling—homesick, longing for the familiar, bored, put upon—while real and even explainable, are most likely stemming from the addicted brain.

This new way of eating is working—too well. Your appetite switch is turning off—and your addicted brain doesn't like it.

Without realizing it, you probably got comfort from almost all your eating, not just from the obvious sweets or starches. A large meal, prolonged eating, these also brought you relief.

Now that your appetite switch is turning off and your meals are becoming smaller and not lasting as long, they are giving you less of a hit of comforting brain chemicals. Thus you are experiencing very subtle withdrawal.

When the addicted brain doesn't get its fix, it starts to tug on you, giving you a variety of thoughts and feelings with one object—to get you to abandon your new program so that you'll come back and take care of it. This isn't an all-out tantrum like a two-year old in the checkout line. It's far more subtle and harder to catch.

If you think an addicted brain couldn't be so powerful that it could seduce you away from your best path, look at any elderly smoker. They cough, they are bent over with their effort to breathe, they could even be carting around a breathing apparatus. And they'll knock you over if you are in their way as they flee a public building in order to smoke. You may have even thought, "I can't believe they're smoking, when it is clearly hurting them."

Their addicted brain has controlled them despite the misery and the doctor visits. Yours has that same degree of power over your eating.

The thoughts an addicted brain sends you seem logical until you pull back a bit and look at the larger picture. The addiction doesn't want you to do that. It wants you to stay a little bit detached from yourself, not quite plugged into your feelings, not quite tuned in to your inner experience. The addiction really wants to interrupt your inner eye.

Your Inner Eye

This is the part of yourself that notices you. It notices what you are doing and why. It catches your patterns. It helps you to know yourself.

I was listening to my foster daughter as she was telling me something important about her week. And for a moment I was distracted by how pretty a picture she made in her new spring dress on the couch with my cat snuggled next to her, all four feet straight out to the side. I thought of getting my camera, but then I noticed I was distracted.

By noticing I was distracted I was able to realize that what she needed was for me to take her in fully and be present to her experience. So I brought myself back, providing an authentic presence as she worked through a problem.

Had my inner eye not been watching, I might have actually

interrupted her to get my camera—my need, not hers—at a most inappropriate time. I would have let her down when she was trusting me to show up for her.

Your inner eye can tell you you're acting snippy cause you're actually mad, that you're ruminating about putting off lunch in order to eat more at dinner, and that your low-lying agitation is actually anxiety about being late for a meeting. Instead of being driven by a craving, you can notice that you have a craving, and then decide how to help yourself with it.

Your inner eye catches on to acts that your thinking brain hasn't caught up to. When you pause to bring a thought into greater consciousness, or center yourself, or journal, or talk to your safest friend, you give your inner eye a chance to tell you what's going on.

You've already been helping your inner eye by pausing every hour to check your stress level and your other felt needs. The more you develop the skill of noticing yourself, the more conscious you can be about what is taking you toward your best goals and what is side-tracking you.

So, what do you notice about yourself now, right now?

Are you centered and connected with yourself, or are you running from yourself?

If you're running, what is it you're running from—a thought? Is that thought about now or about the future or past? If it's about the future or past, you can use the exercise in Chapter 14 to come back to the present.

Are you running from a feeling?

If it's a feeling, make room inside yourself for it. Don't fight it. Allow it.

What do you notice?

How does it feel to be more conscious of what's happening inside you—better, worse, or about the same?

25 Week 4, The Seduction of Stress

Norepinephrine stimulates your lateral hypothalamus.

Say what?

Stress activates your binge center.

You have one brilliant body. It knows how to get stress relief. It makes you eat until either serotonin or your pleasure center is activated. These both have the capacity to turn off the alarms in your body and calm you down.

We wouldn't stress ourselves on purpose, would we? We wouldn't make ourselves do too much, work too hard, demand too much of ourselves—just so we could eat. Would we?

We would. That addicted brain is tricky. If you get real busy, neglect yourself, and activate stress chemicals, that can be the first step in triggering your addictive eating.

Norepinephrine (NE) is the neurotransmitter that completes the link, and when we are exposed to prolonged stress, the actual number of NE receptors in the binge center can increase. Over time this creates an almost automatic reaction of eating in response to stress.

Serotonin soothes NE. By increasing your tryptophan (Test 3), you have already struck a blow for peace. If you analyzed your Test 3 results (in Appendix D), you know exactly just how effective serotonin was. Those results told you whether or not it is important for you to make Change 3.

> **Change 3**
>
> - Eat every 2 or 3 hours.
> - To be counted as a legitimate meal, you must eat some protein.
> - To be counted as a legal snack, it must be 50% protein and 50% complex carb. It must *not* have:
>   a. Wheat
>   b. Sugar
>   c. Flour
>   d. Artificial sweetener (except stevia)
>   e. Msg
>   f. Simple carbs
> - Eat at least 12 units of tryptophan weekly. (That's 4 units a day for three days.)
> - Any time your stress level increases, add 4 units of tryptophan to that week.
> - If you notice you are hungrier, continue to add units of tryptophan until your hunger resumes a normal level.

The following tools will further reduce stress and lower the stress chemicals in your body. Take the pre-test, then proceed though the relief tools, practicing at least three of them.

Your willingness to use relief tools may depend on your addicted brain. That sly scalawag won't want you to reduce your stress chemicals.

It will interrupt your efforts with thoughts such as, "I'll rest just as soon as I get this impossible job done." "I can't stop now. I'm on duty until there's world peace." "I was just about to sit down and then I remembered that I'd better clean all the cat boxes, fence the yard, paint the living room, whip up some costumes for Halloween, wrap my holiday presents, wallpaper the bedroom, and enter the local Martha Stewart look-alike contest."

Turn on your Inner Eye and notice what interrupts the process of lowering your level of stress. If it's just impossible to get around to it, you may have to go to Test 5 in the next chapter, and come back here when you're on the other side of the wall.

Test 4 A—Current Level of Stress--Pretest

Rate the following categories on a continuum from 0 to 5.

Statement	No	Slightly	Mildly	Yes	Very	Severely
	0	1	2	3	4	5
I'm feeling agitated.						
I'm anxious.						
My body is tight.						
I'm tense.						
I'm calm.						
I'm relaxed						
I'm at ease.						
I feel good.						

Relief Tools

Use the following tools in the order given. In other words, start with centering, then use the fear-shrinking protocol, the sacred bowl and, if needed, proceed to metaphorical anger.

Centering

Sit in a way that allows your body to be well-supported, so that your spine is in alignment. Go through the following process, taking plenty of time with each step.

> ✧ Drop your awareness to your feet. Notice your connection with the earth, as the earth grounds you through your feet and through

your contact with the chair or floor.

- ⬥ Bring your awareness up through your body, noticing if any muscle needs to be stretched or repositioned.
- ⬥ Notice your breathing in and breathing out—how your upper body lengthens as you inhale and how you settle into yourself when you exhale.
- ⬥ Take as much time as you need to connect with yourself.

Fear-shrinking Protocol

If you are feeling anxious or worried, use the protocol in Chapter 14.

Becoming Curious[8]
Adapted from Systems-Centered Training

I'm surprised at how uncomfortable I get when I'm at the edge of the unknown. I particularly notice it when I've let go of a familiar state of being, such as being anxious or picking on myself or wanting people to view me in a certain way. There's an emptiness where that comfortable old shoe has been.

Most of us do get anxious when we let go of the familiar, even if the familiar has been making us miserable for years. We are, without our old standby, at the edge of the unknown. We look over the brink and it looks empty. We can't see what's next.

To help ourselves not turn around and run right back to that familiar self-criticism, melancholy, or misery, we can change the dynamic by becoming curious.

Are you curious about what will happen, now that you have let go of that thing? Are you curious about what you will feel, where you will go,

---

[8] The full exercises/protocols are in *the Systems-centered Training Manual.* Go to www.systemscentered.com for more information.

what you will think of?

Notice how you feel now that you are curious. Do you feel better, worse, or the same?

Sacred Bowl

The base of your body is a sacred bowl. It holds your root. Between your root and your heart is your sacred inner self, the energies that hold your direction, your way.

When we shut off our feelings, we block our awareness of the sacred bowl. Learning to use your sacred bowl to hold your feelings puts you back into touch with your inner wisdom. You can then notice what direction your energy wants to go and you will know your best path at any given time.

To open your bowl, take plenty of time with each step:

- ✧ Center
- ✧ Notice if you are holding tightness anywhere in your body. That tightness is a wall against your feelings.
- ✧ Decide if you want to find out what is trapped behind the wall.
- ✧ If you do, either dissolve the wall with warm softness or go through the wall to the trapped feelings.
- ✧ Allow your inner experience to fill the bowl. Let the bowl expand large enough to hold your experience.
- ✧ Notice if any tightness starts to sneak back in. If so, deliberately relax and soften it.
- ✧ Stay with yourself. Continue to notice. Are you curious about what you'll discover as you make room for the experiences in your sacred bowl?
- ✧ How do you feel now that you've made room for yourself?
- ✧ What did you learn?

Metaphorical Anger

When you make room in yourself, you may discover that you are angry about something.

You may have trouble admitting to anger. You are not alone.

If food addicts have one fault that nearly all share, it's that they are too generous. They will, as a rule, give far too much of themselves to others. One of the ways they do this is by turning themselves inside out before they'll let anyone know they are angry.

They'll criticize themselves, they'll get depressed, they'll lose their energy, they'll sacrifice themselves, they'll assume a victim role, they'll do even more for the other person, rather than express their anger directly.

> Food addicts tend to turn anger against themselves.

But anger will always out. It will come out in retaliation, gossip, snide remarks, passive aggression, martyrdom, subtle meanness, a really big explosion (sometimes toward someone who didn't cause the problem), or self-targeting (directing the anger against themselves).

Anger is a very metaphorical emotion and the important thing is to let the metaphor play itself out as a metaphor. The least important thing, surprisingly, is expressing the angry energy to the other person.

I'm going to tell you a story about this, to show you how long anger can affect us and how rapidly the problems it causes can be fixed if you allow the metaphor to be expressed.

For my entire adult life, I've been terrified of public appearances—TV, radio, giving speeches to large gatherings. This is an inconvenient problem for an author with bestselling books that generate speaking invitations for conferences and with media. As soon as I accepted an invitation to speak somewhere, a part of my body would become frantic and

I didn't truly take a relieved breath until it was over.

Despite forty years of experience as a therapist, it did not occur to me to take this to my consultant until I was booked to appear on a TV magazine show. It was one of those problems that both took over my life and seemed invisible, not accepted exactly but as much a part of me as my ease in the water.

My supremely skilled consultant took me through a process that opened a memory. I was back in 7th grade reading class. My regular teacher was sick so a substitute was there. She had given an assignment in which each child was to perform some talent.

I was, at the time, in love with the piano. After a year of lessons when I was about six, I had continued to play, teaching myself by playing lots of music. We didn't have a piano so I asked the teacher if I could come in before and after school and during recess to practice on the piano in her room. She agreed.

We were to perform our talents on Thursday and Friday. Halfway through the class on Thursday, no one volunteered. She asked and no child raised a hand to show their talent. So I said, "I'll go, but I'm not ready so if I don't do well, I want to go again tomorrow."

The teacher said, "All right," waved me up and I played, and I made some mistakes. I wasn't worried because I'd be able to redeem myself the next day. I thought we had an agreement.

That afternoon I practiced hard and knew I was ready. The next day, when everyone was through, I raised my hand, "I'd like to go now. I'm ready."

The teacher waved me away and said with irritation, "You've already gone, Anne."

I was mortified. I would not be able to redeem my mistakes in front of the class. I was so ashamed and humiliated, I wouldn't touch a piano for many years. The piano I'd learned on and had loved, at my grandmother's house, I now blamed. I walked by it every time I visited and sent it a dark glance as if it had been the cause of my humiliation.

The next time I had to perform anything publicly was the viola solo for the High School music concert in the big auditorium my senior year. My mother, who sat back of the middle aisle, said she could see my knees shaking from there.

In one afternoon, I went from being easy with sharing my gifts to a talent recluse. With few exceptions, whenever I had to go in front of a crowd, a critic, or an examining board, I would get so fearful that I'd wish a disaster would befall me so I couldn't go. Once I had a root canal the day after giving a presentation to a hospital staff. I told the dentist, and I wasn't kidding, "I am so glad to be here. This is much better than what I had to do yesterday." (It made her day. It was the first time anyone was happy to get a root canal.)

My consultant continued leading me through the process and I came to a place of realizing I felt angry at the teacher. From my perspective, she had reneged on a contract and she'd been unattuned with a sensitive child. You may be tempted to present her side of the story, but when it comes to releasing anger, it's important to stay with your side of the story. (Two people, two perspectives, two sets of feelings.)

I wanted to mash her ears, to flatten her mouth. I let that metaphor play out. I let my hands mash her ears and press her mouth flat. I let them make those motions as energetically as they wanted to. Suddenly, a door opened that had been locked so long the keyhole had rusted. I felt energy release and flood my body. I could suddenly think of the TV appearance without paralyzing fear.

When I was a girl, I knew nothing about making room for anger. By the time I was twelve I had no skills for expressing or even being aware of my anger. It had been trained out of me when I was a small child.

As it will, my anger had found a way out—toward the innocent piano and into a near-phobia of being noticed. And despite those many years of dormancy, discovering, allowing, and expressing the anger freed me. I did this in a containing environment with my consultant and I advise the same context for you, to start exploration of your own anger in the safe room of a professional therapist.

Notice I didn't have to confront the teacher, who is probably now in that great PTA in the sky. And notice the metaphor of the anger. Mashing the ears that had heard but hadn't listened, flattening the mouth that had spoken irritation. To flatten her the way I had been flattened, to mash her the way my risk and willingness had been mashed.

When we allow angry metaphors to express themselves, we always discover the wisdom of the body. The body knows what was done to it and it knows, with a wisdom we can't make up, what metaphors will both release the harm and express the heart of the injury.

The Process for Discovering the Metaphor
If at all possible, do this work in the containing environment of a professional therapist.

Step 1. Notice indicators that you are angry about something. Common signs:
- Targeting yourself
- Losing energy
- Going from ok to hopeless very suddenly
- Being angry at some innocent party or object
- Being outraged about something

- Getting extra compulsive about something
- Being mean to yourself
- Thinking about eating
- Feeling victimized
- Abandoning plans that would have delighted you for activities that will make you feel worse

Step 2. Center yourself. Relax into knowing what is bothering you.

Step 3. If you can detect the cause, begin talking or writing about it. Tell your safe person about it.

Step 4. Pay very close attention to the metaphors you are using, and then see how it applies to what happened to you.

Examples:

I'd like to shake him. (How were you shaken?)

I wanna kill him. (What was killed for you?)

I could punch him in the mouth? (Were you silenced? Did you take a punch?)

Step 6. Let your expressiveness evolve, continuing to make room for your energy and to notice the pictures or phrases that are coming to you.

Step 7. Giving yourself plenty of room and plenty of time, continue to use your inner eye to follow your process.

Step 8. Afterwards, notice what has changed for you. Notice your energy, your mood, where your attention goes now.

Step 9. Ask yourself, do you feel better, worse, or the same.

Current Level of Stress—Post-test

Now that you have practiced any of the tools that are relevant to your current experience, take the following test again. Rate the following statements on a continuum from 0 to 5. Place a mark in the appropriate box.

Statement	No 0	Slightly 1	Mildly 2	Yes 3	Very 4	Severely 5
I'm feeling agitated.						
I'm anxious.						
My body is tight.						
I'm tense.						
I'm calm.						
I'm relaxed						
I'm at ease.						
I feel good.						

Evaluating your Test 4 Scores

Look at your pre-test and post-test side-by-side.

Draw a line through the marks from top to bottom. Put an arrow at the bottom of the line.

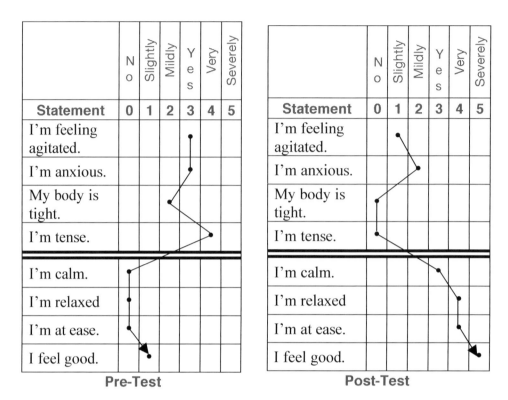

An improvement from using the tools can be seen in the following patterns:

✧ The arrow portion of the line is generally more toward the right than the line connecting the upper dots. (Heading more in a southeasterly direction below the double line as compared to the portion above the line.)

✧ Total the numbers above the line and then below the line in each test. Compare the sums. For example: Pre-test Above—12, Below—1. Post-test Above—3, Below—16. Decreasing sums above the line and increasing sums below the line indicate a decrease in stress.

Use the appropriate tools in this chapter whenever stress is causing you to eat or to forget to sustain the changes that have been working for you. Reducing stress will lower NE stimulation of your appetite switch.

> **Test 4**
> - Eat every 2 or 3 hours.
> - To be counted as a legitimate meal, you must eat some protein.
> - To be counted as a legal snack, it must be 50% protein and 50% complex carb. It must *not* have:
>   - Wheat
>   - Sugar
>   - Flour
>   - Artificial sweetener (except stevia)
>   - Msg
>   - Simple carbs
> - Eat at least 12 units of tryptophan weekly. (That's 4 units a day for three days.)
> - Any time your stress or hunger levels increase, add 4 units of tryptophan to that week.
> - Use at least one stress reduction tool once a day.

26 The Wall

It's as though there is a great wall that never ends and on one side of that wall is the addiction. On the other side is recovery or sobriety.

When I am using, the wall looks very tall. I can't imagine ever getting to the other side. Whatever food I'm holding on to seems precious, impossible to live without.

I resist changing my situation. I tell myself stories. I'm not really addicted, I simply like it. It doesn't really hurt me. I can just eat it now and then. I can make rules about it. I can control it.

No matter how many times it has defeated me, I still have the belief that I can make some compromise that will allow me to continue eating it.

I fight tooth and tongue. I put off doing anything about it. I have lots of excuses. It's not the right time. I need to wait until this other thing is over. I can't afford to be discombobulated. I don't have time. I'm too busy.

I have the persistent belief that I will somehow be much worse off without this food to cling to. Despite these thoughts and this belief, I deny that I am addicted.

And, then, I cross the wall. I let go of the food. I go through withdrawal. I'm hard to live with for a few days. My perceptions are off. I lose my keys and my phone on the same day.

And then, suddenly, I'm on the other side of the wall.

I'm clear-eyed. I'm feeling free. I feel unencumbered. I can't believe how much clearer my mind is. I'm thinking faster. I'm seeing more.

My entire life seems more manageable, not just eating, but nearly everything. I'm appreciating more the beauty in my world. I'm enjoying my people more, letting them in more deeply. I'm feeling my love for my humans and my furry creatures more tangibly

I seem to have more time. I have more energy. I feel better. I wonder, what was the fuss about. This is so much better, here on the other side of the wall.

But I notice, the wall is much shorter on this side. It would be very easy to climb it and drop to the other side. Very easy. Too easy. I'd better not get too close to the wall.

The Addiction

The addiction—it inhabits a part of your brain. It will always be there. It has its fingers into nearly every other part of your brain—your thinking, your feeling, your memory, your perceptions, your values, your priorities, and, of course, your eating. Eating is its fuel, essential for keeping the addiction alive.

We come now to the last test. With this test you go over the wall and find out what it's like on the other side. This will take 4 leaps.

Leap 1. Running start

Leap 2. Jumping over the Wall

Leap 3. Tumbling down the other side

Leap 4. Finding your new balance

Test 5

Test 5 involves letting go of one category of food that triggers your appetite switch. When we've eliminated the other major causes of a faulty appetite switch—peptides, bouncing blood sugar, serotonin, stress—what's left are the chemicals that promote and sustain the addiction.

These are dopamine and certain endorphins, and they are so powerful in the pleasure center of the brain that not even serotonin can stop them. The longer the addiction has been running you, the more powerful the addiction gets, with more and more wires into more and more parts of the brain. All these cells require a frequent bath in the chemicals that soothe and comfort them and when they don't get that bath, they poke at you until you feed them.

They poke first with sabotaging thoughts and ideas, and then they move into hard core cravings. Once you've given in and fed them the foods they want, then they keep you eating more. They make it hard for you to stop eating. They make it impossible for you to eat addictive foods moderately. Their motto is, "More is Never Enough."

There is only one way to get the pleasure center to stop controlling your life. That way is to get abstinent from those foods that trigger the pleasure chemicals. Abstinence is to food addicts what sobriety is to alcoholics. It's the equivalent of being clean and sober.

Unfortunately, we have multiple categories that can trigger us: sweet, starch, fat, starch and fat, sweet and fat, salty, salty and fat, and sweet, fat, and salty. Some of us are addicted to all those categories.

Then there's chocolate, which is almost its own food group to food addicts—having, usually, not only sweet, salt, and fat, but theobromide as well—sedative of the gods.

Unless you go into treatment or assiduously go to 12-step meetings and work the program most thoroughly, it is very hard to get abstinent from all the categories at once.

It's more realistic to get yourself unhooked from one category at a time or even the most potent part of one category.

For example, a good starting place is with obvious sweets, such as desserts, candy, cookies, ice cream, jelly, cake, pie, corn syrup of any kind, and sugar. Isn't that enough to challenge yourself with?

You may already be scared, just from reading that list. So, just sit with it a bit and I'll keep talking.

If that list scares you, you probably are a food addict, and sweets are probably one of the food categories that matter to you a lot. If so, you are on the side of the wall, a very high wall, where life without sweets is hard to imagine. You know instinctively that this sounds like a very difficult challenge.

I can say, from the other side, that it is as bad as you think, but not for very long. Once withdrawal is over, it gets so much easier, that you'll wonder why you waited so long. The benefits roll in abundantly.

So take some time, but don't stop the process. Continue with your first four changes, and get used to the idea that you can go through something that will liberate you in a way you can barely imagine from this side.

I'll tell you how to get ready. I'll tell you what to expect. And you can do it. You can give yourself 3 weeks on this test and see what the difference is for you.

After three weeks, you can decide if you like the peace and clarity so much that you are willing to continue to learn how to live over there, or you can choose to come back.

In any case, do keep the first four changes going. They will still help your appetite switch be more manageable.

Running Start

First you have to decide what food category you'll use for your test. For it to be a true test, it's important that you pick the food category that has your number one drug and trigger food.

Some foods trigger you to eat. Some foods are drug foods. They stimulate the pleasure chemicals that give you comfort or relief. Most foods that are trigger foods are also drug foods, but that's not always the case.

For most people, sweets are the most potent trigger and drug foods. For others, starches, particularly breads, hold the top spot. And for some, fat-rich foods are the main event. The longer you are addicted, the more the brain's target shifts from pure sugar to starch-fat combinations.

Look at the following categories and notice which of the three lists pulls you most strongly.

Sweets	Starches	Fats
Candy	Bagels	Butter
Cookies	Biscuits	Cream
Cake	Bread	Fried foods*
Desserts	Pasta	Mayonnaise
Ice cream	Pizza	Peanut butter maybe
Jam, Jelly, syrup	Rolls	Salad dressings
Pie	Scones	Sour cream

*Fried chicken, potato chips, French fries, fried fish, corn chips, etc

Would you be willing to let go of that one list, for at least three weeks?

If so, continue with the running start. If not, give yourself some time and see if you can become willing. One of my recovery friends said once, "My worst day in recovery is better than my best day in the food."

Ponder that.

Before I was abstinent the first time, I could barely conceive of what such a process could be like. I really couldn't imagine a world without sugar in it. But I did know I had lost too much to my food addiction and I didn't want to lose any more. The thing that fixated me was the idea that I'd never have a particular food again. I just couldn't wrap my mind around it.

And the odd thing was, I hardly ever ate that particular food anyhow, but the image of it represented something to me, something about luxury, well-being, being cared for tenderly. My sponsor said, "Can you give it up today?"

I thought about it. "Yes, I can give it up today."

I could manage getting through this one day without that food or without sugar. And that made the concept work for me.

So, if it seems really difficult to give up your favorite food list, can you imagine getting through one day without those foods? That's all you have to do.

Are you willing to take a running start?

Give yourself a really good chance by preparing to cross the wall.

Step 1. Pick the food list you will start with.

Step 2. Get those foods out of the house. Avoid exposure to them.

Get them out of your desk, your own office, your purse, your car, and get rid of any wrappers or empty containers.

It's important to create safety zones for yourself, to reduce exposure to those items. Plan to avoid any places that feature those foods, particularly your favorite places to eat or obtain them.

 ♦ Do not volunteer to provide any of the foods on your abstinence list for anyone. Don't be baking cookies for the Little League or fruitcake for the priest.

- ❖ Plan to avoid food courts, all-you-can-eat places, buffets, bakeries, and pot lucks.
- ❖ Don't buy, carry, deliver, or handle your trigger foods for anyone.
- ❖ Avoid magazines, TV shows, and cook books that feature lots of trigger foods.

Step 3. Ask your safest, kindest friend if she will support you through this for three weeks.

Ask her if she would be willing to talk, email, or text with you at least twice a day the first week and daily the second and third weeks.

If she's a really super, wonderful, queen-of-the-planet friend, ask if she'd be willing to read Chapters 20-24 in *Lick It! Fix Her Appetite Switch*. (Chapters 18 and 19 are also helpful.) This will give her a full explanation of food addiction and practical ways she can help you.

Step 4. Get real about who in your family is capable of helping you and who won't be able to do it.

I had the fantasy my boyfriend, deep in the cups himself, and my mother, a devoted food addict, would support me. They wanted what was best for me, right? Wrong. They didn't want an interruption in their routines with me.

What a fight ensued when I said I was tired of cooking and would like to take Sunday nights off from making home meals. I know, it's hard to believe the author of *Boundaries* was ever in that situation, but, hey, that was BR, Before Recovery, and where do you think I got the material for *Boundaries* anyway?

I actually cooked two sets of meals for awhile, mine and his, and frankly, I don't know how I stayed abstinent under those conditions. I did have my terrific 12-step friends, two excellent meetings a week, and a sponsor I talked to every day. (And that boyfriend is now ancient history.)

But I don't recommend you cook double. It's better for your brain if you see, smell, and handle only the foods that are on your OK list. Otherwise, some of the other appetite chemicals will gang up with the addictive brain and try to get you back into the fold.

Do tell the truth to yourself about the family members who have the capacity to support you. Don't go looking for diamonds in a coal bin. Most likely candidates are relatives who are:

- Naturally kind
- Not practicing an active addiction
- Can make room in themselves for someone to be on a different path than they are
- Can support without taking over

People who loved me most dearly could not necessarily be a good support to me. Some had their own type of addiction that kept them avoidant to some degree, and learning about my addiction was too much information. Some didn't have the imagination that let them understand what sugar-free actually means. Others wanted to help by bringing me diet ideas or telling me about magic pills.

Remember that most of the people in the world, including many health care professionals, still know very little about the appetite switch. They still cling to the same tool that hasn't worked for at least 150 years—a diet. OK, it works for 5% of the dieting population who are able to sustain their weight loss for longer than 5 years. But 95% of that same population can't sustain either the diet or the maintenance plan for way less than five years.

And except for cell phones, we generally don't keep using tools that only work 5% of the time. Your fridge, if it worked 5% of the time, would be rotten. Your plumbing, working 5% of the time, an obstruction. Your electricity—that better be a short book.

Nope, as tolerant as humans can be about electronic foibles, on the whole, we expect our tools to work more than 5% of the time. But for some strange reason, we accept dieting and continue to promote it, despite its very poor success rate.

So, most of the people you know have this blind spot. Therefore, they are very likely to mention the D-word if you tell them what you are doing. Be ready for that, and don't be derailed by general ignorance.

Here are some snappy comebacks:

"This isn't a diet, Dad. I'm training myself to change the way I eat. Will you support me?"

"I have heard of that raw beets diet, but I'm doing something different. It's a scientific process that turns off my appetite. I'm learning to help my brain make good choices. I hope you won't try to sabotage me now that I've found something that works for me."

"I'm turning off my appetite switch. I found out that was why I've been overeating. It's already working. Are you willing to support me?"

"If you truly want to help, there's a book that will tell you exactly what you can do."

Step 5. Consider investigating a 12-step organization like OA, FAA, EAA, or CEA.

Even if all you do is go to online meetings and listen, you will be inspired. It helps to enter the world of other people who have already been through this.

Step 6. Prepare for withdrawal

Get ready for your brain to object to abstinence. Put some stress-reduction plans in action now.

- ◆ Make spare copies of your keys. Put them in lots of places—purse, desk drawer, glove compartment, best friend's pocket.
- ◆ Copy everything in your billfold—driver's license, credit cards, insurance cards, etc.
- ◆ Make copies of your calendar or schedule for the next month
- ◆ Copy all the phone numbers on your cell phone. The cell phone store can do this or it can be done with your computer or online with some phones. Make a paper copy of these numbers if possible.
- ◆ Consider buying a locator—a little gizmo that can find your purse, cell phone, wallet, and keys.
- ◆ Consider joining AAA or any road service that can rescue your keys from a locked car.
- ◆ Plan to make no important decisions for the next few weeks.
- ◆ Make sure all your snack foods are replenished.
- ◆ Lay in a good supply of foods on your OK list.
- ◆ Check with your doctor if a reduction in blood sugar is going to require modification of any of your medications.
- ◆ Buy grapefruit if you can tolerate it. (It helps with withdrawal.)

All right. You're ready.

FAQ

Q Are you serious? If I give up my sweets for three weeks, I can eat them again?

A Of course. It's your choice. And, once you're in the land of recovery, you might not want to come back to this place where a substance is controlling you and making you miserable.

Q If I'm only going to do this for three weeks, why do it at all?

A Lots of reasons.

- ✧ It is a test. It lets you know for a fact that you are addicted and that pleasure chemicals are a cause of your stuck appetite switch.
- ✧ You can find out two important things:
  - That you can get to the other side
  - What it's like on the other side

It's hard to imagine certain things until you experience them for yourself. Sobriety is one of those. As long as you are eating your drug foods, you are under the influence and can't really assess life without the drug.

Q My church counts on me to make the Dotted Swiss muffins for the Adultery Survivor's Fundraiser. I think I should put Test 5 off till after that event.

A That kind of thought comes from the addicted brain. Would your church support your prolonging something that is unhealthy for you?

Q My husband likes to eat ice cream every evening and he likes for me to sit with him. I hate to change something he enjoys so much. Will it really hurt for me to sit there with him once I start abstinence?

A Exposing yourself to ice cream early in abstinence is a relapse waiting to happen. Not only will your pleasure chemicals get excited, NPY will also make you want it. How long does it take for your husband to eat his ice cream? 10 minutes? Tell him you'll sit with him for ten minutes after he's finished eating (and after he's rinsed his dish in the sink).

Q He likes me to dish it up.

A Is he capable of dishing it up?

Q My sister loves me a lot and I love her. We get together once a month to shop and have lunch. We always go to a bakery that has a café. You said not to go to bakeries. Will it hurt this one time?

A Yes. Bakery cafés always have enticing smells and displays. These will stimulate both your addicted brain and your NPY. Your brain will say something like, "This one little treat won't hurt anything," and you'll be back on the addicted side of the wall before you can blink. Your sister loves you. Tell her you want to keep the ritual, but change the lunch venue. Go to a safe place for lunch. You can blame your lunch needs on me. Your relationship is strong enough to stand a change of restaurant.

Q Should I tell everyone I'm doing this?

A Tell the kind, trustworthy people you can count on being on your side. Do not tell the gossips, the passive aggressive people, the meanies, the slick saboteurs, or the manipulators. Don't tell people who are actively using any sort of drug. Don't tell your binge buddies who count on your participation unless they have already indicated they want to challenge their own addiction right now. (Sometimes people say, "I'll have to do something about that," without meaning they plan to take any real action before the next solar eclipse that's immediately above Northbrook, Illinois.)

Q Why would anyone want to sabotage me?

A You may not be able to imagine just how threatening it will be if you get abstinent while they are still using, even if you make perfectly clear this is something you're doing for yourself and not anything they have to change.

Q   This scares me. I'm afraid I'll lose people who matter to me.

A   Are you saying if they eat pies and you eat pickles it will ruin your relationship? Most people draw back if they think someone will try to convert them. I remember how obnoxious I was after I stopped smoking. I wanted everyone I knew to stop smoking too. We've all been bitten by an evangelizer, of one thing or another. Once they get used to your new ways and trust that you won't pressure them to do likewise, they'll be ok.

Jumping Over the Wall

This is the day you start your abstinence. You'll refrain from all foods on your list. You'll not have a smidge, a taste, one bite, no part of any of those foods. The first day won't be terrible unless you're refraining from the fat-rich foods list. Fat withdrawal starts right away for most people.

You only have to not eat those foods today. Can you get through this one day without those foods?

You might feel as if something is missing or as if you forgot to do something.

Daily To-Do List

- Call your friend
- Eat your snacks
- Eat your meals
- Eat grapefruit if you can
- At the end of your last meal for the day, eat some fruit
- Eat 4 food units of tryptophan at least 5 days this week

FAQ

Q I keep thinking about the next holiday. I can't imagine _____ [holiday] without _____ [food].

A Just think about today. You just have to get through today without it.

Q I can't even imagine getting through today.

A Can you get through the next minute without that food? There are periods when we have to take it a minute at a time.

Q I keep thinking if I just have one bite I'll feel better.

A You can't take just one bite. One bite will be the start of many bites. And you'll only feel better for awhile. You just have to get through the next five minutes, and then the next five minutes. Before long, you'll feel a lot better.

Q I want to go weigh myself.

A Your experience may feel similar to a diet and it's triggering a diet mentality. "If I'm suffering, I must be losing weight." This is a slippery slope back to the other side of the wall. If you haven't lost any weight by tomorrow, you might think, "What's the use. I might as well eat." This is the kind of logic you get with a brain in withdrawal. Remember, this is not a diet. You are fixing your appetite switch.

Q I think I'm eating too much of other things.

A That happens. Your brain is trying to get a fix from other foods. If you are becoming abstinent from sugar and eating a lot of starch (or vice versa), this will probably give your brain what it wants. Don't worry about it. You have only one task today, and that's to be abstinent from the food list you already chose. Later on you can learn about expanding abstinence and how to go about it. But not today.

Tumbling Down the Other Side of the Wall

This is the part where your brain has a fit. This is withdrawal. The most important thing to remember about withdrawal is that it's temporary. It goes away.

For most people, withdrawal is a bear—not a cuddly, furry bed ornament, but a raging separated-from-her-cubs long-clawed beast. It's this way for three to five days. It gives you very powerful cravings, makes you confused, and just a tad irritable—as in make that sound one more time and I'll sit on your head.

Cravings can be like being hit sideways by a tidal wave. You may not always even know what it is you want, just that you need something, real bad and real soon. They steal your focus. They make you forget what you were doing. They make you read the same page over and over as if the words were in Sanskrit.

You may find yourself mindlessly staring into the refrigerator or looking through the cabinets. Weren't you smart to get those foods out of the house?

Now you know why diets couldn't work. Any diet that tried to moderate your drug foods—or take them away—without adequate preparation and without giving you enough information, was setting you up for unexplained withdrawal. Most people go off most diets in three to five days, exactly when the worst withdrawal typically hits.

When a diet tells people to eat only protein for the first two weeks with an occasional vegetable or fruit, it is creating abstinence. However, when sweets or starches are re-introduced, with the goal of moderating them—no food addict can keep that going. It's a set-up for any food addict.

I've worked with many people as they go through withdrawal and here's how sneaky the addiction is. Every once in a while, a person has an easy withdrawal. So then, the addicted brain plants the thought, "Oh, you weren't *really* addicted. You can eat whatever you want."

Now why would the brain even say that if it weren't addicted? Some of those with easy withdrawals went back to the food, got all the same losses, got ensnared again, and then, once more went for abstinence. More power to them. That next abstinence was a bear. The withdrawal showed its claws.

So, if you have an easy withdrawal, thank your lucky stars, but don't be fooled. If your brain starts having sneaky thoughts, that's the addiction. That's your withdrawal.

The Course of Withdrawal

Day 1. I seem to have misplaced something.

Day 2. I'm a bit disoriented. Now and then, food pictures come from nowhere.

Day 3. I'm very distracted. I want my food. I want it. I think I should drive by that food source. Get out of my way.

Day 4. Tie me to the mast. You people are annoying.

Day 5. Tie me tightly. You are on my last nerve.

Day 6. That wasn't so bad. Oh, there's a food picture. I want it, bad. I'm OK. That was easy. I want it, bad. Nothing to it. I think I'll read. I want it, bad. Hmm, withdrawal is a piece of cake. Cake. I want some cake. Oh yeah, I'm OK. It was simple. I'll never eat sweets again. I'm safe. Safe. Safeway. Safeway has lots of sweets. Maybe I'll start dating again. Dating. Dates. Dates and coconut. I'm a nut. Nuts, pecans, almonds. Nope, I'll never overeat again. I'm fine. Fine. Fine-grained. Grain.

Day 7. Sunny with occasional showers.

From then on, the struggle gets much easier day by day. Physical withdrawal continues for about another two weeks, characterized by periods of complete disappearance of symptoms interspersed with occasional really intense cravings, and a fair frequency of sneaky thoughts about various foods or restaurants.

Course of Withdrawal

Intensity	Day 1	Day 2	Day 3	Day 4	Day 5	Day 6	Day 7
Very Strong							
Strong							
Medium							
Mild							
Neutral							

What surprised me about my own withdrawal is how intense a craving could be in one moment—so intense that all I could think about was getting into the car and going to a store—and then how it could disappear so abruptly that I'd forget the craving was even there. And it would go back and forth like that—intense, more intense, severely intense, and then gone.

A Wave of Withdrawal

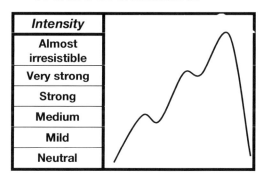

No matter how much you try to convince yourself that you aren't addicted to food, withdrawal is the proof. The addicted brain cells put up a severe fight to get you to eat those drug foods again.

FAQ

Q I had a really easy withdrawal. I don't think I'm addicted.

A Are you willing to wait two more weeks? If so, notice what happens with your appetite over the next weeks. In fact, by charting at least 4 days, you can compare your pattern now with the pattern of your eating after Test 3. Just by eyeballing the two sets of charts what do you notice? Is there a difference in the degree of spikes; are your appetite ratings generally lower? Do they have a low wave-like pattern now? Has the chain eating at the end of the day disappeared? Is there a difference?

Any improvement in your appetite and eating rows indicates that Test 5 is making a difference. Knowing that, do you still want to throw it out? (A strong desire to throw it out when you can see an improvement comes from an addicted brain.)

Q Withdrawal is making me miserable. I can't even think straight.

A I promise you it will pass. Meanwhile, this might be a good time to check out those online meetings. It really helps when you don't try to do it alone.

Q My withdrawal hit me hard on Day 1.

A It does that sometimes. I showed you the average course for sugar and starch withdrawal, but, of course, every body is different and has its own unique process.

Q I'm withdrawing from fats. What will be different?

A   Withdrawal is likely to hit right away and the cravings for fried things will be strong. It is very important for you to eat all your other food, all meals and snacks. You might find yourself eating extra, trying hard to get that old familiar feeling. Eventually it'll sink in that nothing is going to give you that drugged feeling.

   I also found that a time came when I was satisfied with substitutes that had no charm at all while I was using. For example, at a garage sale I discovered a little microwave potato chip maker that used no fat. For 50 cents I gave it a try.

It was wonderful. I got the full potato taste, the crisp, the crunch, and no hit—no hit of pleasure chemicals because there was no oil.

While I was still using, this would have held no appeal (no pun intended). A baked potato chip? What's the point? But in abstinence, it tastes good and is enough.

Q   I don't know if I can make it.

A   Remember that you just have to get through the next 5 minutes without that food. Can you do that?

   You have almost completed the entire system for turning off your appetite switch. And the hardest part is nearly over. Once you've made it through withdrawal, you've done the hardest thing you'll have to do with regard to that ole switch.

   I find some comfort in knowing the hardest part is over. If I can manage that, I can manage whatever is next.

Finding Your Balance

Congratulations. You are on the other side of the wall. Now give yourself a chance to feel your way into this new territory.

Look around. Are colors brighter? Are you more aware? Are you thinking more clearly?

As you get accustomed to being here, notice all the changes. You might even want to make note of them on your chart, just so you can remember what a difference abstinence makes.

Later, as this becomes your new normal, you may forget just how unique an experience this is and value it less. It may seem less special, and you may wander dangerously close to the wall, which is quite easy to fall over, and quite hard to re-climb.

Pay lots of attention. Notice the differences.

Once your brain settles down, notice your appetite switch. You might even chart for four days after your second week of abstinence to see the difference in your appetite and hunger levels now that you've turned off all the major appetite drivers. (Analysis for Test 5 is in Appendix E.)

Welcome to a world where your appetite switch isn't driving you. Meals end. You go on to something else. You have much more time now that your head isn't filled with food thoughts.

If that isn't the case, if you are still plagued by cravings, if you are still eating too much, (and you are sustaining your other necessary changes), then something else on the drug food list is keeping this going.

You decide if you want to repeat test 5 with another food category. If you choose to go over another wall, go back to the beginning of this chapter and take all the leaps again.

Some people do better if they wait awhile before tackling another food group; others have momentum and want to get the whole thing over with. The more support you have, the more bearable it is to scale the wall again.

I found that once I'd given up sugar, I was more willing to let go of other foods. Sugar abstinence taught me I could do it, that I could survive it, and that my life was categorically better without it.

I didn't begin to truly travel my own life path or head toward my own life missions until I started living in recovery. And then, good entered my life at an astounding pace.

Basic Data--Test 5												Circle Wake-up Time									Date			
	Time of Day	5	6	7	8	9	10	11	12	**1**	**2**	**3**	**4**	**5**	**6**	**7**	**8**	**9**	10	11	12	1	2	3	4
Appetite	Can't stop																								
	More food																								
	Craving food																								
	Food focused																								
	Quiet																								
Hunger	Starved																								
	Strong																								
	Moderate																								
	Mild																								
	Not hungry																								
Eating	Protein																								
	Comp carb																								
	Simp carb																								
	Fat/oil																								
Tryptophan-1 dot/unit																									
Caffeine	Yes																								
Satiety	Not satisfied																								
	Satisfied																								
Sress	High																								
	Medium																								
	Low																								
	None																								
Mark the following items just once each day. You can use a mark or make a note for your answer.																									
Sleep Problems				Felt like exercising.							Yes				No	Clarity of thought.									
Gifts of Abstinence:																									

Your Other Choice

It's your body and it's your life. You decide if you want to convert Test 5 into Change 5. If you do, you get to enjoy the fruits of abstinence and to discover that recovery is a gift that keeps on giving. The longer you live over here on this side of the wall, the easier it gets, the more routine.

The addicted brain will visit you occasionally, checking to see if it can pull you back in. It'll give you an occasional craving, especially when you are stressed or feeling difficult feelings. It'll give you the odd idea—such as, you are now capable of making your famous dessert for the Unwed Father's Bake Sale. (You're safer to avoid the entire occasion.)

Change 5

1. Eat every 2 or 3 hours.
2. To be counted as a legitimate meal, you must eat some protein.
3. To be counted as a legal snack, it must be 50% protein and 50% complex carb. It must *not* have:
   a. Wheat
   b. Sugar
   c. Flour
   d. Artificial sweetener (except stevia)
   e. Msg
   f. Simple carbs
4. Eat at least 12 units of tryptophan weekly. (That's 4 units a day for three days.)
5. Any time your stress or hunger levels increase, add 4 units of tryptophan to that week.
6. Use at least one stress reduction tool once a day.
7. Maintain abstinence from the drug and trigger foods you have chosen to release.

The first year will present challenges as you learn how to make it through each holiday and each social occasion without your drug foods. After the first year it becomes second nature. That food will have nothing to do with you. Most of the time you won't even notice it.

(For a completely abstinent Thanksgiving menu and recipes, look at the back of *Lick It! Fix Her Appetite Switch*.

FAQ

Q Suddenly I'm noticing the flavors of the food I'm eating. I'm afraid this will make me eat too much.

A The opposite is more likely. Truth is, most of us food addicts don't really taste the food we're eating until we're abstinent. We're mainlining it as quickly as we can. Most of us do something else while eating—watching TV, reading, working. It's all about getting the fix.

Now that you are tasting your food, you're more likely to notice when satiety kicks in and your interest has left the table.

Q I think I should go back and eliminate the other food categories right away.

A Sometimes it's really hard to tell if that thought is coming from the recovery brain or the addicted brain. If you are still being harassed by cravings, maybe so. Cravings are a pain and a threat when they continue for too long, so letting go of enough trigger food to calm cravings is a positive step. You may need a larger abstinence before they'll leave you alone.

On the other lobe, getting obsessed about restricting yourself is probably the addiction. In that restricted world, you're vulnerable to thinking not eating is good, dropping your snacks, and throwing out meals. Your brain may be enticing you into another compulsion or another big project so you'll get overwhelmed and cave.

This is one of the issues that another recovering person can help you with. Be sure it's someone who can let you pursue your own best abstinence, without pushing you into taking on the abstinence that works for her.

Q I'm feeling reluctant to be with people on eating occasions.

A   Trust yourself here. It may be too soon for you to expose yourself to food displays. You can always join folks after they are through eating.

Q   I have to go to my niece's wedding. I love her and she'd be devastated if I weren't there. But the food. Oy vey!

A   Go to the wedding. Make a separate choice about the reception. If you want very much to be there too, go with a safe, trusted friend. Decide your food strategy before you get there. Will she get your food for you? Tell her what's on your list of OK food. If it's a sit-down dinner, she can field the starch things so that you don't have to pass them. Leave the table during dessert. (I find large catered affairs are happy to provide an attractive bowl of fresh, unsweetened fruit if I ask.)

Q   I don't think I'll ever eat sugar again. (I hear Scarlet O'Hara's voice saying this.)

A   If I had to pick the one thing I've heard the most from clients who were hours away from a relapse, it is the statement, "I'll never eat sugar (or whatever) again." Whether it's complacency, the addicted brain's camouflage, or forgetting the reality of powerlessness, this is one of the two most dangerous thoughts you can have.

The other is, "That won't bother me," with regard to going to a dangerous restaurant, allowing yourself to sit there while someone swoons over your former drug food, or smelling a drug food for longer than 5 seconds.

27 Maintaining Mastery of Your Appetite Switch

You can have a peaceful appetite for the rest of your life. Simply maintain the changes you've proved to yourself work in turning it off.

For two months, you've been focused on this process. Now, as you turn your thoughts in other directions, life will sweep you along. It might distract you from the routines you've established.

If you see your appetite increasing, that's a sign some chemical is out of balance. Run down your list of changes and see which one has been neglected.

Most of the time, when we are dropping some part of our program, it's because something is bothering us. We are getting too close to the wall. Use the tools in Chapter 25, talk to your trusted friend, and get back in touch with your inner eye. Your inner self knows what's wrong.

Remember, appetite switch mastery comes courtesy of the following changes—snacking correctly, tryptophan replacement, stress reduction, and abstinence. And these are a product of replenishing your supplies, planning ahead, and getting timely support.

It actually can be simple. It may not always be easy, but the longer you practice these principles, the more natural it becomes, a way of life in which you are free to pursue your very unique and singular mission.

Appendices

A	*What Next?*	*185*
B	*Analyzing Test 1*	*188*
C	*Analysis of Test 2*	*203*
D	*Analysis of Test 3*	*212*
E	*Analysis of Test 5*	*223*
F	*Resources*	*226*
G	*Index*	*229*
	About Anne Katherine	*232*

A What Next?

After you've made the changes that let you master your eating, where do you go next? I encourage you to live with those five changes for a good long while. Give them a chance to become automatic. Once your body has adjusted to abstinence and your meals automatically become smaller, it is likely your weight will gradually decrease.

If you feel you absolutely must diet, be sure to pick a diet that supports your set of changes. Not all diets will fit your profile and some will actively undo all the progress you've made. Unfortunately, some well-known diet programs will allow or, surprisingly, encourage you to eat foods and chemicals that will fire up your appetite switch and even make your body resistant to weight loss.

A good resource for you is the book *How to Make Almost Any Diet Work*. It rates the main categories of diet programs so that you can pick one that fits your profile, and it tells how to modify diets to fit your profile exactly. It also warns against the greatest danger of dieting—the dread diet mentality that can catapult you into practices that will turn your appetite switch back on.

Listed below is a guide you can use to locate the topics that will support you through your next steps. (Ignore the charts and chart examples in *How to Make Almost Any Diet Work.* Those are much more complicated and use a different food tracking system than the one you learned here.)

Books represented here, all by Anne Katherine:

A—*Anatomy of a Food Addiction*

B—*Boundaries, Where You End and I Begin*

H—*How to Make Almost Any Diet Work*

L—*Lick It! Fix Her Appetite Switch*

M—*When Misery is Company*

W—*Where to Draw the Line*

Guide to Resources

Topic	Description	Book	Page
Abstinence	Sugar	H	214
	Fat	H	340
	Flour	H	218
	Wheat	H	217
Addiction	Science, anatomy, addictive cycle	H	127
	Why some people become addicts	H	129
	Food addiction—types	A	13
	Deprivation	A	48
	Sensitivity to pain	A	44
	Healing	A	95
	A program for recovery	A	115
Boundaries	What they are; how to set them	B	All
	Friendship boundaries	W	116
	Intimacy boundaries	W	137
	Boundary violations	W	77
	Food boundaries	W	266
Dangerous foods	Foods that create a resistance to weight loss	L	38
Diets	Warnings	H	275
	Workable plans	H	283
	How to personalize plans	H	305

Eating disorders	Definitions	H	41
Family	How to handle family food situations	L	107
	The family that sabotages	L	126
Food Addict	Are you one?	H	151
Powerlessness	Blocks to positive action	H	141
Relapse/Slips	How to handle	H	347
Programs	12-Step, anonymous programs—discriminating among them	H	253
Sabotage	Self-sabotage—if you can't get yourself to do what would improve your quality of life	M	All
	Tools for recovery	M	Throughout
Support	Choosing support partners	H	65
	Building a support system	H	81
	Support meeting topics and agendas	H	Chapter ends & appendix A
	Dialogue and skill practice	H	181

B Analyzing Test 1

Your Options

Option 1. If you can tolerate some minimal data analysis and have interest in seeing what the figures show, continue through Appendix B, Part 1, then return to chapter 21.

Option 2. If you love data analysis and you want to learn everything you can about your appetite switch, proceed through Appendix B as far as you want to go.

Part 1.

Gather your seven Basic Data Charts from the Training Week and your seven Test 1 Charts from Week 1. If you have less than seven, but at least four from each week, you can still get some useful information. If you have four Basic charts, then use four Test 1 charts.

Only use Test 1 charts for days you actually had at least four legal meals or legitimate snacks. If you didn't snack on a particular day of Week 1, then that chart can be used as an additional basic data chart. (Cross out the T1 at the top of that chart and make a note so you'll remember.)

Work first with your Basic Data Charts. You will be looking *only* at the Appetite category.

Here's Barry's chart.

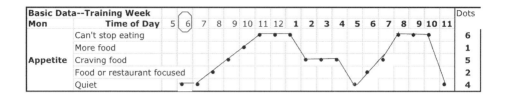

Look at the right end of the chart. The last column is headed by the word 'Dots.' Those numbers are the total number of dots in each row. There are 4 dots in the Quiet row, 2 dots in the Food focused row, 5 in the craving food row, etc.

Step 1. Count the Dots

Now take one of your Basic Data charts. Count the number of dots in the Quiet row and put that number in the dots column in the Quiet row on your Dots Worksheet. Next count the dots in the Food or restaurant focused row on your Data chart. Put the sum in the Food focused row of the worksheet. Continue counting dots for each row and filling in each sum on your Dot Worksheet.

Below you'll see how I've filled in Barry's worksheet.

Your Appetite Dot Worksheet

BD	Dots	Times	Value	Product
Can't Stop		X	5	
More		X	4	
Craving		X	3	
Food focused		X	2	
Quiet		X	1	
Total				

Barry's Dot Worksheet: (Step 1)

BD Monday	Dots	Times	Value	Product
Can't Stop	6	X	5	
More	1	X	4	
Craving	5	X	3	
Food focused	2	X	2	
Quiet	4	X	1	
Total				

Step 2. Multiple the Dots by the Value

Multiply the number of dots in each row by the Value in the 4th column of that row and put the product in the Product column (of that same row).

Barry's Dot Worksheet: (Step 2)

BD Monday	Dots	Times	Value	Product
Can't Stop	6	X	5	30
More	1	X	4	4
Craving	5	X	3	15
Food focused	2	X	2	4
Quiet	4	X	1	4
Total				

Step 3. Total the Product column.

Total the numbers in the shaded Product column.

Your Appetite Switch

Barry's Dot Worksheet: (Step 3)

BD Monday	Dots	Times	Value	Product
Can't Stop	6	X	5	30
More	1	X	4	4
Craving	5	X	3	15
Food focused	2	X	2	4
Quiet	4	X	1	4
Total				57

Follow the same procedure for each Basic Data Chart. Here is a Basic Data Dot worksheet you can make copies of.

BD	Dots	Times	Value	Product
Can't Stop		X	5	
More		X	4	
Craving		X	3	
Food focused		X	2	
Quiet		X	1	
Total				

Step 4. Follow the same procedure for each of your Test 1 charts.

Test 1 Worksheet

T1	Dots	Times	Value	Product
Can't Stop		X	5	
More		X	4	
Craving		X	3	
Food focused		X	2	
Quiet		X	1	
Total				

Step 5. Compile your totals from each week.

Transfer each total from the dark shaded box to the correct cell on the Dots Summary.

Your Dots Summary

Day	Tr. Week Basic Data	Week 1 Test 1			
1					
2					
3					
4					
5					
6					
7					
Grand Total					

Barry's Dots Summary

Day	Tr. Week Basic Data	Week 1 Test 1			
1	57	47			
2	49	35			
3	56	43			
4	53	36			
5	60	55			
6					
7					
Grand Total	275	216			

Understanding Your Results

Compare your grand totals from Week 0 and Week 1. A decrease in the total from week 0 to week 1 means that you have improved the functioning of your appetite switch by decreasing the influence of NPY. Any decrease at all in your Test 1 numbers means that this process is working. You are influencing your appetite switch.

You can also eyeball your two sets of charts. Are there less extreme hills and valleys in your Week 1 charts? Are you achieving a quiet appetite more often? On any day you got your snacks in, did you decrease the hours of wanting more food or being unable to stop eating?

Any improvement, any improvement at all, is a very good sign. After untold years of ignoring your body's natural processes, it's already responding to your intelligent intervention. When you think about it, that's pretty amazing.

Let's say you've been skipping meals for 20 years. If after only one week, you are seeing an improvement, that's marvelous.

FAQ

Q   I want the information, but I don't want to have to do the analysis. Will you do it for me?

A   Yes. Go to my website, www.masteryourappetite.com. There is a fee. You must have at least 5 Basic Data charts and 5 Test 1 charts for days you actually snacked and had 3 meals. I can only promise to analyze the charts of the first 400 people who sign up and will only guarantee to provide this service for the first 6 months after the publication date of this book. After those parameters, you can check the website and see what's available.

Q   I just have 3 basic data charts. What does this mean?

A   Hmm. It means you have a very small sample of days to compare your pre-change brain with the subsequent tests you'll be conducting. You might still get some information. If you want to fix this, keep very good daily charts for each subsequent test. With each test, you'll at least have more data from the previous week to compare it to.

Q   If I have 3 Basic Data charts, how many Test 1 charts should I use for comparison?

A   Use 3 Test 1 charts. Barry just kept records for 5 days for week 0, so he used 5 Test 1 charts for his comparison.

Q   I forgot to chart on some of the hours during the day. How do I handle skipped hours?

A   Look at Barry's Basic Data chart for Thursday. He forgot to chart at 9 and 10 AM.

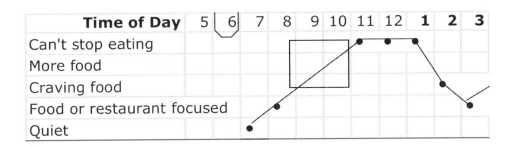

He looked at the cells the line passed through, and counted those as virtual dots. (Look at the small square on the chart in that location. When you count Barry's dots on the More food (shaded) row, he has no dots. But the line passes through that row at 10:00 AM. So it's counted as a dot and you can see that that row has a 1 in the column at the far right.

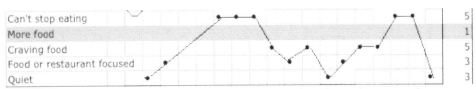

Q   My numbers went up instead of down. What does that mean?

A   That happens sometimes. I wouldn't worry about it. Wait till the end of Test 2 and see what the numbers show. For some people, until their snacks contain protein, their appetite switch won't calm down.

Another cause of increased numbers is an increase in addictive eating. If the addicted brain is having a fit because you are learning this process, it may be pushing you to have more food.

You can see for yourself if this is what's going on. Check your evening eating after you've had dinner on any Test 1 day. If your eating continued despite your snacking, that's the addicted brain calling the shots.

Q   My Test 1 days are uneven. Some days I remembered to snack, some days I didn't. What do I do?

A   Only use the Test 1 charts for the days you snacked and only use the same number of Basic Data charts for comparison. On the bright side, any day you forgot to snack during Week 1, Test 1, you can add those charts to your Basic Data charts.

If your number of Basic Data charts are skimpy, you'll now have more charts you can use to compare to the next two tests.

Q   This whole calculation process made me crazy. I don't want to do it.

A   That's OK. Read the next paragraph and then skip to page 201.

If you lay out your 2 sets of charts side-by-side, can you see a difference? Can you feel a difference? If you can stand it, keep your Test charts just 2 more weeks. After that, you won't need them unless you want to use them to stay conscious. Skip to page 201.

Part 2. Additional Analysis for Inquiring Minds

If you've had it with statistics, go back to chapter 21. I would rather you protected yourself from being overwhelmed than for you to make yourself endure a process you hate.

Otherwise, in this section we'll look at other NPY indicators to see which of your practices are increasing NPY and which ones are decreasing it. You'll need an equal number of Basic Data and Test 1 charts. Remember Test 1 charts are testing the first change, and a T1 chart is to be used only if you actually did make the Test 1 change that day.

NPY Worksheet	BD	Date:							
Definitions: To be counted as a meal it must have protein. To be counted as a snack, it must not have any sugar, flour, wheat, refined starch, msg, or artificial sweetener, except stevia.									
Behavior	Point count	Day 1	2	3	4	5	6	7	Behavior Total
Skipped Breakfast*	15								
Skipped L or D	10								
Delayed Breakfast*	10								
Skipped Snack1	10								
Skipped Snack2	10								
More than 3 hours pass before legal eating	5/hour								
Eating for 2 consecutive hours	10								
Daily Total									
									Grand Total
*A meal or snack gets counted as breakfast only if it occurs within 2 hours of waking up.									

Step 1. Determine the points for each behavior, for each of your Basic Data charts.

Fill in the points on the NPY Worksheet under the appropriate Day column.

Look at your first Basic Data chart. Did you skip breakfast that day? If so, put a 15 in the 1 column. If you delayed breakfast by an hour, put a 10 in the Delayed breakfast column.

Did you skip lunch? Put a 10 in the Skipped L or D column. If you skipped both lunch and dinner, put a 20 in that cell. Skipping either snack costs 10 points apiece. And for every hour that you didn't eat past 3 hours of your previous intake, it's a toll of 5 points per hour. Finally, any time you eat 2 hours in a row, that gets 10 points.

Step 2. Total your points for each day.

Barry's Example

Here's Barry's Day 1, BD Chart and how to rate it.

Barry did a good job of following the instructions about not changing anything about his eating during Training Week (Week 0). He made an accurate representation about how he ordinarily eats.

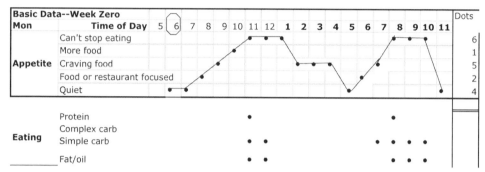

Obviously Barry skipped breakfast. 15 points are entered into the appropriate cell. He had some protein at 11 and 8 so they get counted as lunch and dinner. He saved himself 20 points.

He skipped both snacks, but of course on Week 0, he didn't even know he was supposed to snack. So, again, he did a good job of gathering accurate data, and 10 points per missed snack go on his worksheet.

Barry's BD NPY Worksheet

NPY Worksheet	BD	Date:							
Definitions: To be counted as a meal it must have protein. To be counted as a snack, it must not have any sugar, flour, wheat, refined starch, msg, or artificial sweetener, except stevia.									
Behavior	Day Point count	1	2	3	4	5	6	7	Behavior Total
Skipped Breakfast*	15	15							
Skipped L or D	10								
Delayed Breakfast*	10								
Skipped Snack1	10	10							
Skipped Snack2	10	10							
More than 3 hours pass before legal eating	5/hour	50							
Eating for 2 consecutive hours	10	20							
Daily Total		105							
									Grand Total
*A meal or snack gets counted as breakfast only if it occurs within 2 hours of waking up.									

Every hour of delayed eating past the time breakfast should have occurred is counted at 5 points an hour. If that seems harsh, remember, every hour of delayed eating costs you in terms of NPY production. Barry awakened at 6 and should have eaten no later than 7. From 7 to 11 is 4 hours. That's 20 points.

Since he had lunch at 11, he should have had a snack by 2:00. He ate a legitimate meal at 8. (His eating at 7 was a simple carb so it doesn't get counted either as a meal or snack.) From 2:00 to 8:00 is 6 hours. That costs 30 points. Morning and afternoon added together—of hours passed before legal eating—total to 50 points.

He ate into a second hour at midday and into a second hour after dinner. This costs 10 points for each occurrence. Barry's total for Day 1 is 105.

Step 3. Rate your Test 1 charts in the same way.

Your T1 NPY Worksheet

NPY Worksheet T1 Date:									
Definitions: To be counted as a meal it must have protein. To be counted as a snack, it must not have any sugar, flour, wheat, refined starch, msg, or artificial sweetener, except stevia.									
Behavior	Day Point count	1	2	3	4	5	6	7	**Behavior Total**
Skipped Breakfast*	15								
Skipped L or D	10								
Delayed Breakfast*	10								
Skipped Snack1	10								
Skipped Snack2	10								
More than 3 hours pass before legal eating	5/hour								
Eating for 2 consecutive hours	10								
Daily Total									
									Grand Total
*A meal or snack gets counted as breakfast only if it occurs within 2 hours of waking up.									

Barry's T1 record for the third day.

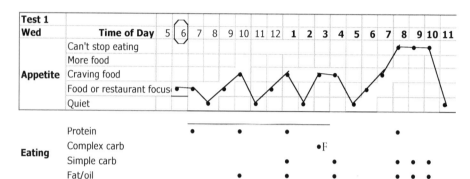

Barry did a great job of adding breakfast and incorporating his snacks. These changes made a noticeable difference. You can see right away that his hills are less steep and he has more valleys.

His records also reveal an issue. Even though he had a legitimate T1 snack at 3:00, he continued to crave food and to eat, and the food he ate at 4 could not be considered a snack. A fruit, without a protein, did not stop his appetite. This tells me Barry has some blood sugar problems and that Test 2 will be important for him.

Dinner should have occurred at 6 since his snack was at 3:00. He delayed dinner by two hours and ate into a second hour twice.

Barry's T1 Worksheet

NPY Worksheet T1 Date:								
Definitions: To be counted as a meal it must have protein. To be counted as a snack, it must not have any sugar, flour, wheat, refined starch, msg, or artificial sweetener, except stevia.								
Behavior	Day Point count	1	2	3	4	5	6	7	Behavior Total
Skipped Breakfast*	15								
Skipped L or D	10								
Delayed Breakfast*	10								
Skipped Snack1	10								
Skipped Snack2	10								
More than 3 hours pass before legal eating	5/hour			10					
Eating for 2 consecutive hours	10			20					
Daily Total				30					
									Grand Total
*A meal or snack gets counted as breakfast only if it occurs within 2 hours of waking up.									

Barry's NPY Analysis

	BD	T1		
NPY Grand Total	515	255		

Comparing his basic data before he made any changes, to his scores after making a simple change, shows he's made a marked improvement in his appetite switch, having turned down his NPY in just one week.

Step 4. Place your totals into the NPY Analysis chart.

Now put both your grand totals here.

	BD	T1		
NPY Grand Total				

Understanding the Results

A decrease in the grand total with the Test 1 change means that NPY was one of the chemicals that was keeping your appetite switch stuck in the on position. You now know two important things:

- ✧ NPY was one of the causes of your overeating.
- ✧ You can fix it by eating three meals and two snacks a day.

Converting Test 1 to Change 1

If Test 1 revealed that NPY was driving your eating, you now know that this is one of the changes that works in calming your appetite. By continuing to follow the Test 1 protocol, and making a commitment to this practice as an ongoing change, you can ensure that your appetite switch will bother you less.

FAQ

Q If I ate lunch but skipped dinner and had no legal intake the rest of the day, how many hours do I count as the interval of not eating?

A Count 3 hours past your latest legal intake and start there. Then count every hour until you go to bed. For example, if you had lunch at noon, your next feeding should have occurred by 3:00. Let's say you retired at 11 pm. Then the interval without eating legal food lasted 8 hours.

> **Change 1**
>
> 1. Eat every 2 or 3 hours.
> 2. To be counted as a legal meal, you must eat some protein.
> 3. To be counted as a legitimate snack, it must *not* have:
>   a. Wheat
>   b. Sugar
>   c. Flour
>   d. Artificial sweetener
>   e. Msg
>   f. Simple carbs

Q My numbers didn't improve all that much. I had a heck of a time adding breakfast.

A Even though Test 1 requires only one change—adding snacks—Test 1 may involve additional changes for people who have been skipping meals. Give yourself some slack in not expecting perfection immediately. Any improvement at all, with the goal firmly in mind, is a good sign.

C Analysis of Test 2

Evaluating your Test 2 charts will operate exactly the same way as the analysis of the Test 1 results, so I won't give you all the gritty details. If you need a reminder, go back to the last appendix.

Part 1. Your Dots Analysis

Step 1. Assemble your T2 charts.

Step 2. Count the dots in each row of the appetite category.

Put the totals for each row in the appropriate cell of column 2 of the Dots Worksheet.

Dots Worksheet

T2	Dots	Times	Value	Product
Can't Stop		X	5	
More		X	4	
Craving		X	3	
Food focused		X	2	
Quiet		X	1	
Total				

Step 3. On each row, multiply the dot total with the Value and put the answer in the Product column.

Step 4. Total the Product column

Step 5. Fill out a Dots Worksheet for each day of Week 2.

Step 6. Transfer your Totals from the Product column to Your Dots Summary for Week 2.

Your Dots Summary from Chapter 21 already has the Week 0 and Week 1 figures on it.

Your Dots Summary

Day	Tr. Week Basic Data	Week 1 Test 1	Week 2 Test 2		
1					
2					
3					
4					
5					
6					
7					
Grand Total					

Step 7. Compare your totals from each of the three weeks.

Understanding Your Results

A decrease in NPY numbers from the previous weeks means two

wonderful things. Your NPY is moving to a back burner, and your PYY is showing up. If your numbers have improved (become smaller), then this tells you to convert Test 2 into Change 2 and to make it a regular part of your daily routine.

> **Change 2**
> 1. Eat every 2 or 3 hours.
> 2. Have at least some protein at every meal.
> 3. Eat two 50-50 snacks a day. They must *not* have:
>   Wheat
>   Sugar
>   Flour
>   Artificial sweetener (except stevia or xylitol)
>   Msg
>   Simple carbs

Part 2. Additional Analysis for Inquiring Minds

(If you've had it with statistics, go back to the chapter you were working with.)

In this section we'll look at both NPY and PYY indicators.

Step 1. Fill out the NPY worksheet using your T2 charts.

You've had experience filling out an NPY worksheet from Appendix B. Determine the points for each behavior, for each of your Test

NPY Worksheet	T2	Date:							
Definitions: To be counted as a meal it must have protein. To be counted as a snack, it must not have any sugar, flour, wheat, refined starch, msg, or artificial sweetener, except stevia.									
	Day	1	2	3	4	5	6	7	
Behavior	Point count								Behavior Total
Skipped Breakfast*	15								
Skipped L or D	10								
Delayed Breakfast*	10								
Skipped Snack1	10								
Skipped Snack2	10								
More than 3 hours pass before legal eating	5/hour								
Eating for 2 consecutive hours	10								
Daily Total									
									Grand Total
*A meal or snack gets counted as breakfast only if it occurs within 2 hours of waking up.									

2 charts. Fill in the points on the NPY Worksheet under the appropriate Day column.

Step 2. Total your points for each day.

Step 3. Place your totals into the NPY Analysis chart, transferring the BD and T1 figures from Chapter 21.

	BD	T1	T2	
NPY Grand Total				

Part 3. PYY Analysis

Assemble your Basic Data charts from Week 0 and your Test 2 charts from Week 2.

Step 1. Taking each Training Week chart, one at a time, enter the point count for each behavior shown on your charts.

For example, if you had breakfast within your first two hours after waking up, give yourself 15 points for that day. Record 10 points if you had a legal snack 2-3 hours after breakfast. Of course, during Training Week, you didn't even know about legal snacks, so the chances are you won't have those points.

The first five measures on the worksheet give credit for the behaviors that balance the appetite peptides in the brain. The last three measures are indicators that your efforts are making a difference.

Did you awaken with an appetite? Look on your Basic Data chart for the hour you woke up. How did you rate your appetite? If it was quiet, you had no appetite. Then no points go into that cell.

A lack of morning appetite means that satiety kicked in for you

PYY Worksheet	BD	Date:							Behavior Total
Legal Snack—50% protein & 50% comp carb									
Day		1	2	3	4	5	6	7	
Behavior	Points								
Ate Breakfast by 2nd hour after waking.	15								
Ate legal snack 2-3 hours past breakfast	10								
Ate meal 2-3 hours past Snack 1	10								
Ate legal snack 2-3 hours past lunch	10								
Ate meal 2-3 hours past snack 2.	10								
Awakened with an appetite	10								
No appetite following legal eating	10/incx								
No eating in hour past legal snack or meal.	10/incx								
Daily Total									
									Grand Total

overnight, when it was of no use to you. You either had delayed satiety, or addictive nighttime eating caused you to still be full or satiated at breakfast time. If you didn't know better, you would skip breakfast and put yourself into another day of peptide-triggered eating.

When PYY is working, your appetite goes away after legal eating. Each time you have a quiet appetite after a meal or legal snack, mark 10 points per incident.

When PYY is working, you won't eat in the hour after a legal snack or meal (unless a food addiction overrules it). For now, since we're only measuring PYY and not the addiction, give yourself 10 points for each time you don't eat in the hour following a legal snack or meal.

Example: Barry's chart

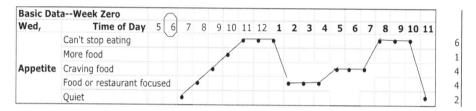

Barry's PYY Work-sheet:

Barry scored a perfect zero. He's following the ideal plan if he wants to keep overeating. His practices are guaranteed to keep his appetite switch on and his PYY asleep.

What a difference after Test 2!

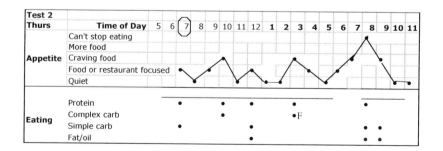

Just by eyeballing the two charts, it's immediately obvious that Barry's appetite switch is becoming regulated.

PYY Worksheet T2 Date:									Behavior Total
Legal Snack--50% protein & 50% complex carb									
Day		1	2	3	4	5	6	7	
Behavior	Point count								
Ate Breakfast by 2nd hour after waking.	15	15							
Ate legal snack 2-3 hours past breakfast	10	10							
Ate meal 2-3 hours past Snack 1	10	10							
Ate legal snack 2-3 hours past lunch	10	10							
Ate meal 2-3 hours past snack 2.	10								
Awakened with an appetite	10	10							
No appetite following legal eating	10/incx	30							
No eating in hour past legal snack or meal.	10/incx	40							
Daily Total		125							

Except for the delay of the evening meal, Barry followed the Test 2 protocol exactly and his points reflect this. He now has a morning appetite, which helps him to eat breakfast. When *you* start waking up with an interest in eating, this is a very good sign. We are supposed to have hunger and appetite in the morning.

Barry's meals and snacks are stopping his appetite, so he isn't eating past his mealtimes, with the exception of dinner. We can't tell from this one chart, whether or not Barry's evening eating is from the addiction or lack of PYY.

By waiting so long to eat, he'd gone an extra two hours past the time his next meal was due. That could well be the cause of his prolonged appetite after dinner and, hence, the additional eating.

It's also possible that the addiction gave him thoughts that made him delay the meal, just so it would have some unchallenged eating once dinner was over. This discrimination will have to wait for Test 5.

Meanwhile, his figures show an amazing improvement in his peptide functioning after just two weeks. Imagine, Barry mistreated his body for 35 years and it is recovering normal appetite function in two weeks. Yea Body!

Step 2. Use your T2 charts to enter points into the PYY Worksheet.

PYY Worksheet	T2	Date:							
Legal Snack—50% protein & 50% comp carb									Behavior Total
Day		1	2	3	4	5	6	7	
Behavior	**Points**								
Ate Breakfast by 2nd hour after waking.	15								
Ate legal snack 2-3 hours past breakfast	10								
Ate meal 2-3 hours past Snack 1	10								
Ate legal snack 2-3 hours past lunch	10								
Ate meal 2-3 hours past snack 2.	10								
Awakened with an appetite	10								
No appetite following legal eating	10/incx								
No eating in hour past legal snack or meal.	10/incx								
Daily Total									
									Grand Total

Step 3. Transfer your grand totals to the Peptide Analysis chart.

Peptide Analysis	BD	T1	T2	
NPY Grand Total				
PYY Grand Total				

Understanding the Results

Improved peptide functioning is revealed by a decrease in the NPY totals and an increase in PYY totals over time.

An increase in the PYY grand total with the Test 2 change means that a lack of PYY has been keeping your appetite switch stuck in the on position. You now know two important things:

- Insufficient PYY was one of the causes of your overeating.
- You can fix it by eating three meals and two 50-50 snacks a day.

> **Change 2**
> 1. Eat every 2 or 3 hours.
> 2. To be counted as a legitimate meal, you must eat some protein.
> 3. To be counted as a legal snack, it must be 50% protein and 50* complex carb. It must *not* have:
>   a. Wheat
>   b. Sugar
>   c. Flour
>   d. Artificial sweetener (except stevia)
>   e. Msg
>   f. Simple carbs

D Analysis of Test 3

Part 1 of Test 3 Data Analysis will operate exactly as in the previous two tests. You'll compare the appetite figures from Test 3 to the figures you've already calculated.

Part 1. Your Dots Analysis—Appetite

Step 1. Assemble your T3 charts.

Step 2. Count the dots in each row of the appetite category.

Put the totals for each row in the appropriate cell of column 2 of the Dots Worksheet.

Dots Worksheet--Appetite

T3	Dots	Times	Value	Product
Can't Stop		X	5	
More		X	4	
Craving		X	3	
Food focused		X	2	
Quiet		X	1	
Total				

Step 3. On each row, multiply the dot total with the Value and put the answer in the Product column.

Step 4. Total the Product column

Step 5. Fill out a Dots Worksheet for each T3 chart.

Step 6. Transfer your Totals from the Product column to Your Dots Summary for Week 3.

Your Dots Summary from Appendix C already has the Training Week, Week 1, and Week 2 figures on it.

Your Dots Summary—Appetite

Day	Tr. Week Basic Data	Week 1 Test 1	Week 2 Test 2	Week 3 Test 3	
1					
2					
3					
4					
5					
6					
7					
Grand Total					

Part 2. Serotonin Post-Test

Circle or fill in the answer.

Question						
Are you now hungry when you wake up?	Yes			No		
At what time of day are you most vulnerable to chain eating now?						
How long does a chain eating episode typically last now? (In hours)	.5	1	1.5	2	2.5	3+
What foods do you eat when you chain eat now? Circle any combination that is typical for you.	Fruit Veg Protein Comp carb.			Sweet Starch Fat Salt		
Have you noticed a relationship between feeling stressed and chain eating?	Yes			No		
When you are stressed, does your chain eating typically increase or decrease?	Decrease			Increase		
How would you rate your average level of stress in the last week?	Low		Med		High	
How vulnerable did you feel the last few days? Was your degree of vulnerability:	Low		Med		High	
How relaxed have you been lately?	Very		Some		Not	
How have you been sleeping?	Soundly		Slightly disturbed		Very disturbed	

Chapter 23 has your Serotonin Pre-test. Compare the two sets of answers. Any shift in answers from the right columns toward the left columns is an improvement.

Part 3. Hunger Analysis

Serotonin decreases hunger as well as appetite. What happened to your hunger level after increasing serotonin? You may already have felt or seen a difference. If not, your charts may know something you don't.

To do the hunger analysis, use 5 charts from the Training week or Week 1. The charts you use must include the eating subcategories. (The first charts of Training Week don't include the info on protein, simple carb, etc.)

Dot Analysis—Hunger

Compile dot information on the hunger rows exactly as you did on the appetite rows.

Part A

Step 1. Assemble your five early charts.

Step 2. Count the dots in each row of the hunger category.

Put the totals for each row in the appropriate cell of column 2 of the Dots Worksheet.

Dots Worksheet—Hunger

Training Week or T1	Dots	Times	Value	Product
Starved		X	5	
Really hungry		X	4	
Moderately hungry		X	3	
Mildly hungry		X	2	
Not hungry		X	1	
Total				

Step 3. On each row, multiply the dot total with the Value and put the answer in the Product column.

Step 4. Total the Product column

Step 5. Fill out a Dots Worksheet for each of your five early charts.

Step 6. Transfer your Totals from the Product column to Your Dots Summary for Week 1.

Part B

Step 1. Assemble your T3 charts.

Step 2. Count the dots in each row of the hunger category.

Put the totals for each row in the appropriate cell of column 2 of the Dots Worksheet.

Dots Worksheet—Hunger

T3	Dots	Times	Value	Product
Starved		X	5	
Really hungry		X	4	
Moderately hungry		X	3	
Mildly hungry		X	2	
Not hungry		X	1	
Total				

Step 3. On each row, multiply the dot total with the Value and put the answer in the Product column.

Step 4. Total the Product column

Step 5. Fill out a Dots Worksheet for each Test 3 chart.

Step 6. Transfer your Totals from the Product column to Your Dots Summary for Week 3.

Your Dots Summary--Hunger

Day	Tr. Week or Week 1	Week 3 Test 3
1		
2		
3		
4		
5		
6		
7		
Grand Total		

Understanding Your Results

A decrease in hunger and appetite numbers means two wonderful things.

- ✧ Your serotonin is being replenished
- ✧ Serotonin is an important factor in turning off your appetite switch.

If your numbers have improved (become smaller), then this tells you to convert Test 3 to Change 3 and make it a regular part of your daily routine.

> **Change 3**
>
> 1. Eat at least 12 units of tryptophan weekly. (That's 4 units a day for three days.)
> 2. Any time your stress level increases, add 4 units of tryptophan to that week.
> 3. If you notice you are hungrier, add units of tryptophan until your hunger resumes a normal level.

Part 4. Stress Analysis for Inquiring Minds

If you've had it with statistics, go back to Chapter 23. Protect yourself from being overwhelmed. For those who like learning more about how their bodies work, continue.

In this section you can find out how increased tryptophan has affected your stress level. You'll need an equal number of T1 and Test 3 charts. Remember Test 3 charts are testing the third change, and a T3 chart is to be used only if you actually had the prescribed number of tryptophan units that week.

Dot Analysis—Stress

Compile dot information on the stress rows exactly as you did on the appetite rows.

Part A

Step 1. Assemble five T1 charts.

Step 2. Count the dots in each row of the stress category. Put the totals for each row in the appropriate cell of column 2 of the Dots

Worksheet.

Dots Worksheet—Stress

T1	Dots	Times	Value	Product
High		X	4	
Medium		X	3	
Low		X	2	
None		X	1	
Total				

Step 3. On each row, multiply the dot total with the Value and put the answer in the Product column.

Step 4. Total the Product column

Step 5. Fill out a Dots Worksheet for each of your five T1 charts.

Step 6. Transfer your Totals from the Product column to Your Dots Summary for Week 1.

Part B—Step 1. Assemble your T3 charts. Fill out a Dots Worksheet for the latter 5 days of Week 3.

Step 2. Count the dots in each row of the stress category. Put the totals for each row in the appropriate cell of column 2 of the Dots Worksheet.

Dots Worksheet—Stress

T3	Dots	Times	Value	Product
High		X	4	
Medium		X	3	
Low		X	2	
None		X	1	
Total				

Step 3. On each row, multiply the dot total with the Value and put the answer in the Product column.

Step 4. Total the Product column

Step 5. Transfer your Totals from the Product column to Your Dots Summary for Week 2.

Your Dots Summary--Stress

Day	Week 1 Test 1	Week 3 Test 3
1		
2		
3		
4		
5		
Grand Total		

Two More Options

If you want even more information, you can compare your patterns of stress eating. By looking at eating or appetite that increases with higher stress levels, you see the direct effect of NE on your appetite.

By noticing when eating turns off your stress, you can see evidence that you have triggered some soothing chemical in order to manage your stress.

Here is an example of such a chart:

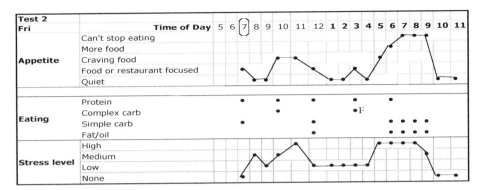

This is Barry's chart from week 2.

He wasn't stressed when he awakened. He had breakfast and left for work. Traffic was so slow he worried he'd be late to work and his stress level increased. Once he got to the office, he was comfortable with his task line-up for the day and his stress decreased as he began working.

At 10:00 he had to go to a meeting, which, in his opinion, was unnecessary and chaired by idiots. Idiot leadership always increases stress.

Lunch included comfort foods, and his stress level dropped until right before he left the office when he found out a co-worker had been fired. His stress level jumped to the roof and stayed up there until he'd had four hours of chain eating.

As soon as his stress level elevated, his appetite also jumped, from a quiet state to craving food. Once he started eating at 6:00, he wanted more food and then couldn't stop eating until his appetite finally turned off at 10 pm. His stress started turning off at 9:00.

This is clear NE caused eating. His chart shows he had his meals and Test 2 snacks at the appropriate intervals. Peptides did not cause this eating. Since he had not yet started Test 3, he also did not have the serotonin buffer that might have mediated the stress to some degree.

He ate until his comfort and pleasure chemicals kicked in, and then those foods and chemicals kept the eating going, even past the time the stress chemicals began fading.

You can look at your charts for the same signs, correlating stress increases with increased eating or appetite. You can also notice what food groups turn off the stress.

Understanding the Results

A decrease in the stress grand total with the Test 3 change means that serotonin has decreased your general level of stress. This, with the other Test 3 results, also confirms that NE (norepinephrine) was affecting your appetite switch.

Improved serotonin functioning is revealed by a decrease in hunger, appetite, and stress totals over time.

Clearly, serotonin is important for turning off your appetite switch.

E Analysis of Test 5

Begin analyzing Test 5 after the 2nd week of abstinence. This allows time for your appetite to settle down.

Part 1. Your Dots Analysis—Appetite

Step 1. Assemble your T5 charts.

Step 2. Count the dots in each row of the appetite category.
Put the totals for each row in the appropriate cell of column 2 of the Dots Worksheet.

Dots Worksheet--Appetite

T5	Dots	Times	Value	Product
Can't Stop		X	5	
More		X	4	
Craving		X	3	
Food focused		X	2	
Quiet		X	1	
Total				

Step 3. On each row, multiply the dot total with the Value and put the answer in the Product column.

Step 4. Total the Product column

Step 5. Fill out a Dots Worksheet for each charted day past the 2nd week of Test 5. (At a minimum, this would be week 6)

Step 6. Transfer your Totals from the Product column to Your Dots Summary for Week 6.

Your Dots Summary from Appendix D already has the Training Week and Weeks 1, 2, and 3 figures on it.

Your Dots Summary—Appetite

Day	Tr. Week Basic Data	Week 1 Test 1	Week 2 Test 2	Week 3 Test 3	Week 6 Test 5
1					
2					
3					
4					
5					
6					
7					
Grand Total					

Part 2

You can duplicate any of the previous analyses if you'd like—comparing hunger or stress data—to discover the impact of abstinence on other aspects of your life.

You can also compare satiety rows from Test 1 to any of the other tests, by simply noting the average hours of satiety Week 1 as compared to the average hours of satiety on any other charted week.

Remember that it's a good sign to be hungry and not satiated upon awakening, and for hunger and appetite to go away after meals and snacks. We aren't looking for a flat line, but small, even hills and valleys.

The biggest indicator of addictive eating is chain eating, particularly in the evening. When you've achieved the optimal level of abstinence from your drug and trigger foods, chain eating should disappear. Reappearance of chain eating means that you've been eating too close to the edge, taking chances with questionable foods, had too much legitimate starch at one sitting, are depleted in serotonin, or are too stressed—or all of the above.

Use some stress reduction tools to find out what's wrong and your willingness is likely to return.

F Resources

Books

Alcoholics Anonymous Big Book, 4th edition
The simple and profound program that initiated recovery for millions of addicts of every kind. 2001

Anatomy of a Food Addiction, Anne Katherine
A program to overcome addictive eating. 1991

Boundaries, Where You End and I Begin, Anne Katherine
Good Boundaries strengthen recovery and provide insurance against relapse. 1991

Eating Mindfully, Susan Albers
Techniques for becoming more mindful about when, how, where, and why you are eating. 2003

Lick It! Fix Her Appetite Switch, Anne Katherine
Humorous, what works, what doesn't, and how to use your influence wisely. 2009

Live Large, Cherie Erdman
Affirmations and actions for loving your body regardless of size or

shape. 2003

The Twelve Steps and Twelve Traditions of Overeaters Anonymous
The twelve steps of recovery as applied to compulsive eating, an adaptation of the original 12 and 12 of AA.

When Misery is Company, Anne Katherine
End self-sabotage and become content. 2004

Where to Draw the Line, Anne Katherine
With every encounter, we either demonstrate that we'll protect what we value or that we'll give ourselves away. 2000

Self-Help Organizations

Compulsive Eaters Anonymous—CEA
www.ceahow.org

Eating Addicts Anonymous—EAA
http://www.eatingaddictionsanonymous.org/
(202) 882-6528

Food Addicts Anonymous—FAA
www.foodaddictsanonymous.org
561-967-3871

Overeaters Anonymous—OA
www.oa.org
505-891-2664

Recommended Professional Organizations

Specialists in treating eating disorders and food addiction:
ACORN Food Dependency Recovery Services
www.foodaddiction.com : 941-378-2122

Food Addiction Institute
http://www.foodaddictioninstitute.org

Gurze Books—specializing in resources for eating disorder recovery
www.gurze.com

International Association of Eating Disorders Professionals
www.iaedp.com
800-800-8126

Milestones In Recovery
http://www.milestonesprogram.org/
800-347-2364

To find therapists who are at the cutting edge of therapeutic effectiveness:
Systems Centered Training
www.systemscentered.com

G Index

1

12 Step Programs · 108–9
12-step organization · 165
1st Weekend · 95

A

Abstinence · 159–61
Addicted Brain · 106–8, 106–8
Addicted to food · 105
Addiction · 157–59
anger · 149
Anonymous programs · 108
Appetite · 19
Appetite biochemicals · 28
Appetite Switch · 1
Athlete Envy · 56
Automatic patterns · 26

B

Balance · 175
Barry · 13, 188, 189, 190, 192, 193, 194, 196, 197, 198, 199, 200, 207, 208, 209, 220
Baseline · 28
Basic Data · 14, 15, 16, 21, 79, 187, 188, 190, 191, 192, 193, 194, 195, 196, 203, 205, 212, 223
Biased perspective · 6
Binge · 75
Binge center · 109, 144
Blood sugar · 74
Blood tests · 2, 8
Boredom · 139
Brain · 105
Brain function layers · 107
Brain Pathways · 96
brain repair program · 23
Brain Trick · 95

C

Caffeine · 51
Centering · 147
Chain eating · 128
Change 3 · 145
Chemical breakdown · 18
Chemical packages · 27
Chemical problem · 4, 8
Clandestine eating · 106
Comfort chemicals · 109
Comfort foods · 104
Complex carbohydrate · 28
Complex carbs · 42
Compulsive Eaters Anonymous · 108, 226
Consumables · 98
Control-group data · 28
Cow · 118
Craving · 14
Curious · 147

D

Daily protocol · 72
Data Analysis · 120
Data Chart · 21
Data Chart 4 · 53
Data Chart Day 1 · 16
Data Chart, Day 3 · 44
Day off · 95
Declaration of Independence · 138
Degrees of hunger · 19
Denial · 140
Depression · 127
Diet · 85
Dieting · 109
Disability · 140
Dopamine · 159
Dreams · 133

E

Eating Addicts Anonymous · 108, 226
Eating for comfort · 66

Endorphins · 159
Exercise · 57

F

Familiar · 138
Family · 163
Famine · 77
Fats · 29
Fear Shrinking Protocol · 89
Five tests · 2, 10, 12
Food Addicts Anonymous · 108, 226
Food as a tool · 103
Food Chart · 42
Food chemicals · 28
Food composition · 42
Force · 58
Forgetting the time · 93
Fork in the road · 11
Friend · 163

G

Good records · 8
Guide—Resources · 184

H

History · 77
Homesick · 138
How to Make Almost Any Diet Work · 108
Hunger · 19
Hunger and appetite · 18
Hungry for affection · 18
Hurry-up mode · 25

I

Inner eye · 142
Insulin · 74
Internal Saboteur · 141

J

Jules · 45
Jumping Over the Wall · 169

L

Lactose intolerant · 133
Leaps · 158
Lose weight · 7, 87

M

Magic Pill · 124
Make room · 140
Martha Stewart · 146
master**your**appetite.com · 51
metaphorical anger · 153
Milk · 42
Mixed grain · 33

N

Negative prediction · 91
Neuropeptide Y · 74
No Skipping · 3
Norepinephrine · 109, 144
NPY · 74, 75–78
NPY vulnerable · 76

O

Old ideas · 7
Oprah · 54
Options · 120
Organizing · 102
Overeaters Anonymous · 226
Overeating · 4, 8

P

Pause and notice · 26
Plan · 85
Planning Place · 83, 88
Pleasure center · 159
Polypeptide YY · 111
Portable Meals · 81
Powerlessness · 109–10, 186
Protein · 28
Proteins · 29
PTSD · 127
Pursuit of Comfort · 126
PYY · 111–13, 114–15

R

Relief chemicals · 109
Relief Tool · 89
Relief Tools · 147
Replacing snacks · 98
Research tool · 3
Rule · 1, 84
Rule 1 · 72, 84
Rule 2 · 6, 85
Running Start · 161

S

Sacred Bowl · 148
Satiety · 62, 114
Self-Observing System · 146
Serotonin · 124–29, 134–35
Serotonin Pre-Test · 128
Serotonin Test · 124
Shooting into the dark · 9
Shopping · 82
Simple carb · 42
Simple carbohydrate · 28
Simple carbs · 38, 40
Snack Planning Tool · 99
Snacks · 86
Snappy comebacks · 165
Starchy vegetable · 33
Stevia · 72
Stress · 66, 144–46
Stress—Post-test · 154
Stress--Pretest · 146
Success · 98
Sugar or starch · 38

T

Test 1 · 72, 84
Test 1 Data Chart · 81
Test 2 · 114, 122
Test 2 Chart · 117
Test 3 · 128, 130
Test 3 Chart · 129
Test 4 · 155
Test 5 · 159
Testing period · 2
Training Week · 3, 6, 7, 10, 20, 187, 197, 205, 212, 213, 214, 223
Tree thumping · 97
Try hard · 109
Tryptophan · 131
Tryptophan Sources · 129
Tryptophan Warning · 132
Tumbling Down · 171

U

Units of Tryptophan · 131
Urine tests · 8

V

Vegetable · 33
Vegetarian · 133
Vicious circle · 4
Vulnerability to pain · 127

W

Warning · 7
Weekly Planning Tool · 100
Weigh and measure · 27
Withdrawal · 166, 159–61
www.master**your**appetite.com · 193

X

Xylitol · 72

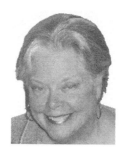

About Anne Katherine MA, CEDS, LMHC

Warm, honest, dedicated, Anne Katherine crawled into recovery from her own food addiction in 1982, and then her life changed. "Recovery created a Great Divide—between the life I led when my brain was in the mothballs of addiction and the explosion of potential that became possible when food was no longer the center of my life. I never would have believed it could make such a difference to find release from the addiction."

From that point forward she became a relentless sleuth on the hunt for the biochemistry of food addiction, trusting that there had to be a biological cause rather than the pat explanations of too lazy or weak-willed. These efforts led to a wealth of cutting edge discoveries including the appetite switch, her popular book, *Anatomy of a Food Addiction,* and to a series of treatment programs, culminating in the Master Your Appetite process.

In addition to forty years of experience as a therapist specializing in eating issues, most of that time in private practice with some years working in or consulting to hospitals, she has an MA in psychology, is a Licensed Mental Health Counselor, and a Certified Eating Disorders Specialist, with recognition from the International Association of Eating Disorders Professionals.

Now retired from private practice, she speaks at conferences, leads retreats, and guides the online Master Your Appetite program. Her companion book is *Lick It! Fix Her Appetite Switch*, for your friends and family members who want to support you.

www.master**your**appetite.com

www.annekatherine.org

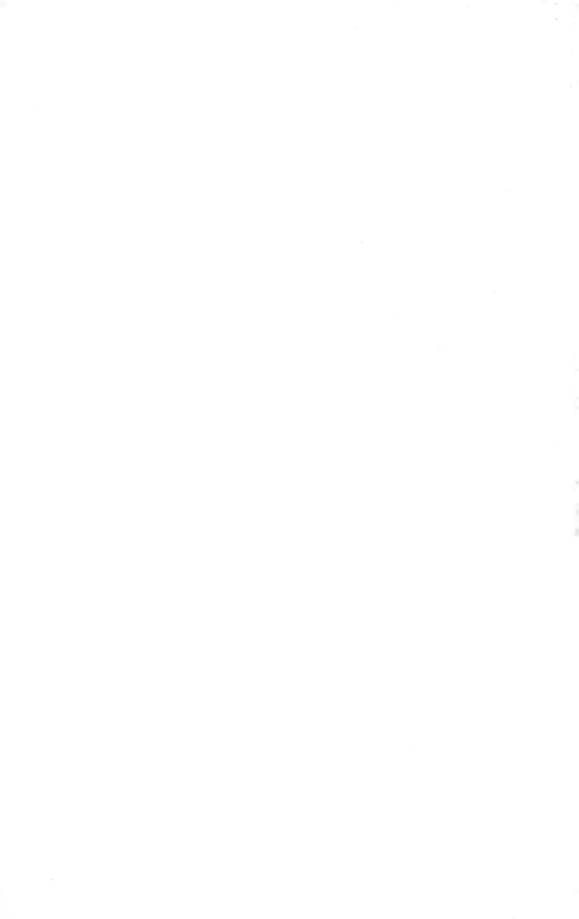

Made in the USA
Lexington, KY
07 November 2010